Your Patient Safety Survival Guide

Your Patient Safety Survival Guide

How to Protect Yourself and Others from Medical Errors

Gretchen LeFever Watson

ROWMAN & LITTLEFIELD
Lanham • Boulder • New York • London

Published by Rowman & Littlefield
A wholly owned subsidiary of
The Rowman & Littlefield Publishing Group, Inc.
4501 Forbes Boulevard, Suite 200, Lanham, Maryland 20706
www.rowman.com

Unit A, Whitacre Mews, 26-34 Stannary Street, London SE11 4AB

British Library Cataloguing in Publication Information Available

Library of Congress Cataloging-in-Publication Data

Names: Watson, Gretchen LeFever, 1960– author.
Title: Patient safety survival guide : how to protect yourself and others
   from medical errors / Gretchen LeFever Watson.
Description: Lanham : Rowman & Littlefield, [2017] | Includes
   bibliographical
   references and index.
Identifiers: LCCN 2017001510 (print) | LCCN 2017003020 (ebook) | ISBN
   9781538102091 (cloth : alk. paper) | ISBN 9781538102107 (electronic)
Subjects: | MESH: Patient Safety | Medical Errors—prevention & control |
   Cross Infection—prevention & control
Classification: LCC R729.8 (print) | LCC R729.8 (ebook) | NLM WX 185 |
   DDC 610.28/9—dc23
LC record available at https://lccn.loc.gov/2017001510

Printed in the United States of America

For Paris Ann
In memory of Dory, Gretchen Osgood, and Bud
Because of Don

Contents

Foreword

About a year ago, I ran into my friend Doug as he headed to visit his mother in the hospital. She was recovering from orthopedic surgery at a world-renowned academic medical center. Doug said Mom would be back on her feet in no time.

Sadly, I could not encourage his confidence. My organization, The Leapfrog Group, issues letter grades rating hospitals on how safe they are for patients, an A, B, C, D, or F on how well they protect patients from errors, injuries, and infections. We tell the truth, even when the truth is uncomfortable.

So I had to be honest with Doug. Despite its storied reputation, his mother's hospital was far worse than average on preventable infections, surgical errors, and never events. We gave the hospital a "C" for safety, up from a "D" a year ago. Families should worry when loved ones are admitted to this hospital.

Doug had a number of good questions. Why would an otherwise stellar hospital allow problems with preventable infections and mistakes? Is there something amiss with the surgeons, the nurses, somebody else? And most importantly, how could his family protect Mom?

I launched into my two-minute elevator speech on patient safety. No, it's not the individual physicians or nurses at fault, it's the culture of the hospital that determines whether patients are safe or not. And even reputable hospitals can have a culture that doesn't truly put patients first. This is why as many as one thousand patients a day die from preventable errors in the United States. And families can literally save patient lives; they should monitor all the medications and watch that caregivers follow the rules, like washing their hands before entering the patient's room. Communities need to hold hospitals accountable.

Doug is one among many people with concerns and questions, and the elevator speech only goes so far. So I was delighted to see my colleague Gretchen LeFever Watson writing this book as a resource for all of us to share. This is an accessible and definitive overview of the key issues in hospital safety, including what families, hospitals, clinicians, and communities can do to protect patients—and help solve this devastating problem.

Gretchen brings an unusual breadth of knowledge and compassion to the subject, having fought for safety from many perspectives. She endured every mother's worst nightmare, an error that nearly killed her four-year-old. She's served in senior roles in health systems, as a community leader in a coalition addressing safety, and as an educator teaching safety to clinicians-to-be, helping the next generation understand how patient experience is shaped not only by their involvement as individual caregivers but also by the culture of the larger health system and community they are a part of.

There is a great deal of important information in this book, useful for caregivers, leaders, patients, and advocates alike. But fundamentally Gretchen is an optimist with the soul of a healer, so the book is more inspiration than criticism. And more than anything else, improving safety requires such inspiration. Safety is about putting the patient first every minute of every day, washing hands every time, carefully honoring rules for inserting needles or administering medications, even when you are in a hurry or tired or in a bad mood. The patient is always first priority. It takes inspiration to never for even one minute forget why that matters and what's at stake.

Some hospitals with deep endowments and soaring reputations can fail to make the grade on safety. Conversely, some hospitals with mundane reputations, serving marginalized communities, achieve some of our highest ratings for safety. What makes the difference is not money or fame but the humble art of putting the patient first.

The good news about Doug's mom: over the past year her hospital finally embraced that humble art, and just last month Leapfrog upgraded their Hospital Safety Grade to an "A." The bad news for Doug's mom: this happened too late for her. She suffered surgical errors and painful infections, causing debilitation for her and the family over many hard months.

Someday all hospitals will earn an A, and our families will not have to endure unnecessary suffering like Doug's family did. This book will guide us there, and inspire us to persevere.

Leah Binder, President & CEO
The Leapfrog Group
November 29, 2016

Acknowledgments

The message of this book represents a culmination of a long series of professional and personal experiences, beginning with a year abroad as a US Junior Ambassador of Goodwill through the Rotary Exchange Program. As a seventeen-year-old with no prior exposure to German, I learned to speak the language proficiently and see the world differently—ever after appreciating that "languaging" affects perceptions and behavior.

In terms of early influences for this book, I'd like to thank Professor Fredric Sugarman for raising the bar on my career aspirations and encouraging me years ago to apply to Boston University (BU), where I learned to think critically and recognized that great scholars are willing to mentor ordinary students and citizens who strive to bring their lofty ideas into meaningful practice, as the late professors Philip Kubzansky and Sigmund Koch did for me. BU is also where my friend Jonathan Knee introduced me to ideas of the likes of Alasdair MacIntyre (then visiting professor at BU), whose philosophical writings from decades ago still inform the field of patient safety and medical malpractice. And BU is where Professor Emeritus Frances Grossman and her graduate students—especially Suad Noah and William Pollock—brought research and the field of clinical psychology to life for me.

My graduate school selection was based purely on the amount of financial support offered, but it turned out that attending the University of Illinois at Chicago (UIC) was a great choice. The program honored the Boulder scientist–practitioner model of clinical psychology, and my dissertation advisor, Brian Vaughn, encouraged his students to pursue high-quality projects that could be completed in a feasible amount of time—getting us out of the program faster than its then eight-year average. Because my UIC funding required that I simultaneously pursue clinical psychology (study of abnormal development) with developmental psychology (study of normal development), the program molded me as an academic boundary spanner—something that has always served my career well. My postdoctoral training at Georgetown University Medical Center reinforced the value of the Boulder Model and cross-disciplinary investigations.

My first professional job was with the Naval Hospital in San Diego, where I learned how much one's social community could affect one's quality of life. Professionally, I grew up fastest at Eastern Virginia Medical School (EVMS). It was at EVMS where Larry Pickering, MD, encouraged me—at the time a shy and timid full-time clinical faculty member—to pursue a research project that mattered to me, which, in turn, altered the course of my career. It was also there where Ardythe Morrow, PhD, mentored me in epidemiology research, public health practice, and academic publishing. I am also grateful to Children's Hospital of The King's Daughters, an EVMS affiliate, for having provided funding and support for me to lead the formation of a school health coalition—a 10-year endeavor that shaped my appreciation for the need to more directly involve the public in the fight against common medical mistakes.

I am not able to name Sentara Healthcare patients, executives, employees, and affiliates who inspired me to write this book. You know who you are.

I might never have had the idea of writing a book if I had not met psychiatrist Sally Satel. Sally arranged for me to spend parts of several summers working out of the American Enterprise Institute and introduced me to Jo Ann Miller—an accomplished editor and champion of aspiring authors. Upon learning about my desire to write a patient safety book, Jo Ann offered sound advice on preparing a winning proposal and encouraged me to obtain a position with relevance to the field on a national level. The situation did not allow Jo Ann to edit the manuscript for this book; however, a national platform opportunity did materialize. I took it, which, indeed, turned out to be important for writing this book.

While working with and for Mike Summers, provost at Tidewater Community College in Virginia Beach, to create a workforce to support the rapid adoption of electronic health record systems across the country, he patiently allowed me to focus on how the project could impact patient safety. Two people who were especially important in this regard are Leah Binder, President & CEO of The Leapfrog Group, and Dr. David Classen, a physician, technology innovator, and academician with a passion to improve patient safety. Leah and David, as well as partners and staff at Pascal Metrics, graciously shared their time and expertise and encouraged me to continue to pursue my ideas about improving the human side of safety. Gratitude also goes to patient safety experts who answered my calls and emails without knowing me, including Drs. Atul Gawande, Albert Wu, Vikki Entwistle, Kathleen Leonhardt, and John Clarke.

The most significant contributor to this book is Andrea Powell Arcona, PhD. Andrea was my first clinical practicum student who grew to become a cherished colleague and friend. We collaborated for over twenty years, and Andrea spent many hours discussing this book and helped shape its premise and cowrote an earlier version of chapter 3. Perhaps had it not been for her booming clinical practice and wonderfully busy family life, this book would have been better through her ongoing contributions.

Some critical influences on my thoughts about patient safety have been more obtuse. My sister Cynthia spent most of her Boston College freshman year in Brigham and Women's Hospital, where I visited her almost every day. The Bernard Lown Cardiovascular Group, whose patient care philosophy was revolutionary at the time, treated her. Because of their approach, Cynthia is alive and healthy today, and I was exposed as a young adult to what was the best hospital care America had (and might still have) to offer. Every step of the way, Cynthia's care was guided both by science and compassion and delivered in a manner that instilled hope while adhering to the notion of "nothing about me without me." Learning decades later that one of her cardiologists formed the Lown Institute to protect patients from unnecessary diagnosis, treatment, and harm has again been comforting—this time it affirmed the direction of many of my past and present professional pursuits.

On a more pragmatic level, my mother managed to always ask how the book was coming along without a whiff of that dreaded maternal tone of "Is-your-room-clean-yet?"

A former colleague and a few friends rallied around me for a moment of good cheer as I embarked on what seemed like the daunting task of writing a book: Sid and Wendy Vaughn, Mo and Mona Ghobriel, and Rick and Kathy Fee. Having celebrated that start of the process with them kept me from giving in to any thought about quitting.

A number of colleagues and friends stood by me through various highs and lows that formed the background of experiences that led up to publishing this book; I know I would not have survived with my spirit equally intact without their support, including my kindred spirit Mary Hull, Mary Wong, Thursday Groups of Encinitas, Steve and Melanie Smith, Trisa Thompson, Brenda Gruber, Joe and Nancy Francis, Lynn Zoll, Linda Owen, Irv Wells, Linda Frantz, Carla Galanides, Marlyn Fabrizio, Michele Bordelon, Kim Hron-Stewart, Keila Dawson, Bob Frenck, Glen Snyders, Jeanne Lenzer, Sue Parry, Lou Lloyd-Zannini, Fred Ernst, Bob Whitaker, Jonathan Leo, Shannon Brownlee, Aubrey Blumsohn, Nancy Oliverie, Kevin Martingayle, Joe Bouchard, Eileen Chiccotelli, Roy and Vivienne Phelps, Jeff Hammaker, Bob and Carol Bibbs, Larry and Betsy Leonard, Don and Susan Bradway, Lorraine Jordana, Julie Seipel, Katie Taylor, Sel and Liz Harris, Dan Evans and other dear KGPC family and friends. There were also my PEO Sisters, two aunts who included me in their nightly novenas, a family priest, six Lake Woebegon–like siblings, fun-loving aunts and uncles, cousins, academic mentors and collaborators Drs. David Antonuccio (who I consider a treasured friend and extraordinary clinical psychologist and defender of academic integrity), David Healy, Linda Perloff, Gershon Berkson, Christopher Keyes, Arnold Sameroff, Ron Seifer, Leslie Feil, and Margo Villers, and a few anonymous guardians who provided unsolicited financial support at a critical life juncture.

Suzanne Staszak-Silva, executive editor at Rowman & Littlefield, has earned my eternal gratitude for taking a chance on me as a first-time book author. This book would not have been possible without the ever-ready staff, particularly Kathryn Knigge and Elaine McGarraugh.

While working on the book, my windsurfing friend Pam Levy introduced me to Vin Altruda, former president of Borders Group, who, in turn, introduced me to other publishing pros, including Jill Tewsley and Mary Jo Zazueta—working without an agent, their just-in-time guidance and services were invaluable. The same is true of my author friend and fellow psychologist Lindsay Gibson. I'd also like to thank Lynn Garson (attorney and author of *Southern Vapors*) for always being at the ready with publishing advice and support. If outside graphic designers were allowed, the kind, competent, and creative Kami Hines of Hines Designs stood ready to assist with the book jacket design.

My heartfelt appreciation goes to my daughter, Paris Ann, for surviving, for tolerating years of ridiculously long conversations about my work, and for reading most of this manuscript before I sent it to the publisher. Of course, I am forever grateful to my husband, Don, for enduring all the hours I spent holed up in my study and for keeping me grounded during the writing process. Without his patience, support, and pragmatic wisdom, I might not have finished this book.

Introduction

Healthcare is a dangerous business. Every day, over one thousand hospital patients in the United States die and many more are needlessly harmed by the care they receive. When I was a young mother listening to doctors at a military hospital apologize for nearly killing my four-year-old daughter, I had no idea how often human error jeopardized our health and safety. And it wasn't until fifteen years later, after being hired to serve as the director of patient safety and performance excellence for a large healthcare system, that I realized our country was in the midst of a patient safety crisis.

Since taking that first patient safety job, I have learned much about the science and practice of safety in hospitals and nursing homes; as well as in nuclear power plants, shipbuilding and ship-repair facilities, and motor repair shops. One thing is clear: every industry is doing a better job with safety than the healthcare industry, but none is working harder to improve it.

The public first got a glimpse into the world of patient safety in 1999, when the Institute of Medicine (IOM) published the now seminal report titled *To Err Is Human*. Until then, healthcare had never systematically tallied and publicly reported how often care that is supposed to help and heal patients actually harms them. The report claimed that nearly one hundred thousand US hospital patients died each year as a result of medical mistakes. This finding shocked people inside and outside of the industry.

Since *To Err Is Human* was published, a great deal has been done to improve patient safety. Hospitals have started to model themselves after other high-risk industries that manage to maintain stellar safety records. Companies that experience less than one in a million disasters, in spite of their high-risk operations, are referred to as high reliability organizations, or HROs. Even though most American hospitals now follow the same steps HROs use to build cultures of safety in their facilities, this has not been enough. Through improved monitoring of patient safety events, it has become evident that nearly half a million (or more) hospital patients in the United States die each year as a result of preventable errors—more than twice the rate of harm originally estimated by *To Err Is Human*.

Preventable medical mistakes are now one of the leading causes of death in our country, far ahead of deaths due to auto accidents or almost all diseases that modern medicine seeks to treat. Any other industry that inflicted so much harm on its customers would be declared catastrophically unsafe, and it would be shut down or boycotted altogether. Perhaps it's no wonder that disillusionment or project fatigue have begun to set in among healthcare professionals and that there has been recent Internet chatter about the patient safety movement flickering out. But giving up on patient safety is not an option.

Besides its human toll, this crisis is financially untenable. On an annual basis, patient safety events result in billions of dollars of direct healthcare charges, and about one-quarter of these involve out-of-pocket expenses. Taking into account indirect costs for lost workdays and short-term disability claims, the total outlay for healthcare-induced harm is estimated to be over one trillion dollars annually.

In any given year, all of us are likely to have someone we love be hospitalized, or be hospitalized ourselves—perhaps to deliver a baby, recover from an illness or injury, replace a joint, treat cancer, or repair a cardiac condition. Thus we all have a stake in making hospitals and other healthcare facilities safer. We, the public at large, represent the industry's customer base, and yet the patient safety movement has treated our involvement largely as an afterthought. Getting a handle on any organization's safety always requires employee engagement, which hospitals have sought to address with varying degrees of success. But when it comes to healthcare, consumer engagement is also of paramount importance because the industry's customers become a dynamic part of the system the moment any of us walk or are wheeled through the hospital doors.

To be fair, healthcare has become increasingly sensitive to the need for and benefits of greater patient engagement. Experts now admonish us to speak up for safety. But this amounts to too little too late, especially when our safety instructions are first delivered during the anxiety-ridden hospital experience. It is about as effective telling a child how to behave once he is in the throes of a temper tantrum. Rather than receiving eleventh-hour and generic guidance about our role in safety, we need to be prepared to take specific actions to protect our loved ones and ourselves long before we are confronted with a hospital visit.

Ironically, at this juncture, much of the work that needs to be done to make hospitals safer must take place outside of them, in the communities where we live and work. You might wonder how the public could possibly help make the complex and complicated process of delivering hospital care safer, but we can. In fact, directing public efforts toward preventing just three types of patient safety events could reduce unnecessary hospital deaths considerably—perhaps by as much as 50 percent over a five-year period, which is a national goal that was set in 2000 and that healthcare has never come close to achieving.

Three issues that make sense to immediately tackle through public engagement are hospital-acquired infections, off-the-mark procedures (also called wrong-site surgeries), and medication administration errors. Together, these three categories of harm represent the most prevalent, predictable, and preventable medical mistakes—a trifecta of sorts.

If it seems hard to believe that tackling just these three problems alone could dramatically downshift the magnitude of the crisis, consider the fact that each year one hundred thousand people die from infections that they pick up as a result of their hospital care. That is a sizable portion of all preventable instances of hospital-induced deaths. Medication errors are another leading cause of preventable death in hospitals, with a third of all such errors occurring during the bedside administration of drugs. As a category, off-the-mark procedures don't occur nearly as often as medication errors or hospital-acquired infections; however, every off-the-mark procedure signals, like a bellwether, that something might be seriously wrong with the healthcare delivery system.

Here, though, is what is special about the identified trifecta of safety issues. In addition to being prevalent, predictable, and preventable, these events can be avoided with simple, quick, and essentially cost-free behaviors that are performed during almost every patient encounter and in eyeshot of patients. They are essential and visible routines; however, for a myriad of reasons, providers don't employ them or don't do so consistently. If the public were to realize the use of these habits could mean the difference between life and death, who wouldn't make sure they were employed?

Mastering key safety habits is something every healthcare provider must do, something every patient wants them to do, and something the public can help them do. I learned early in my career as a clinical and pediatric psychologist that changing the behavior of a troubled child is highly dependent upon changing the behavior of the adults around the child. So it goes with patient safety. In order to change the behavior of healthcare providers, we must influence the behavior of the patients around them. But we must also prepare providers to react approvingly when we do catch them having a momentary slip or lapse or the impulse to take a shortcut. In other words, education for the public must be tightly coupled with interventions that target healthcare professionals.

Developing a comprehensive strategy to unite patients and providers around the use of concrete safety habits represents the only realistic way to achieve consistent performance of safety routines that might seem too simple to matter. Community coalitions are a proven method for raising public awareness, motivating civic action, and promoting specific health-related behavioral change across large groups of people and organizations, but they are conspicuously absent from the patient safety movement. A key to their success is the ability to prioritize goals and objectives according to local interests and resources. Building a local patient safety coalition requires considerable and coordinated effort on the part of healthcare organizations, public health practitioners, and diverse community groups—but such work pays dividends. Successfully reducing the current safety trifecta (or any one of its component problems) will build momentum, confidence, and the capacity to tackle other pressing safety issues, including, for example, the American opiate epidemic and related heroin crisis. In the process, our trust that healthcare providers can reliably deliver safe care might be restored.

When things do go wrong, more than anything else, patients and families desire an apology, but the prevailing reaction of hospitals and providers is to deny their mistakes. For patients and families, such dishonesty adds insult to injury. Although medical mistakes are common, instances of reckless negligence are rare. Most medical mistakes involve honest human error, and this is as true for hospitals as it is for most nursing homes, freestanding surgical centers, and outpatient clinics. When a serious mistake happens, the event can be traumatizing for providers, especially if they are unable to be honest about what went wrong. The agony providers carry with them often leads to burnout that, in turn, undermines their ability to offer quality and safe care.

A few trailblazing hospitals and providers have shown us a better way. Their work proves that when hospitals and providers fully disclose adverse events—meaning that they admit their mistakes, learn from them, and apologize for them—everybody benefits. Patients and providers recover more quickly, and the number of malpractice claims, settlement costs, and administrative fees are reduced. Support for this sort of honest and open communication is gaining momentum and legislative backing, but there is still a long way to go.

From personal experience, I know how healing a timely and genuine apology can be. It might have been the only thing that suppressed an otherwise litigious family member's desire to sue the physicians and hospital that harmed my daughter. Fortunately she survived, but far too many families suffer more tragic hospital encounters.

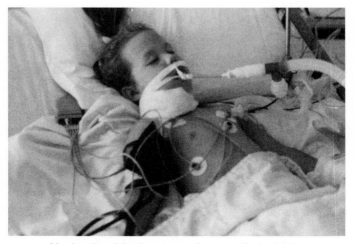

My daughter lying in a coma after a medical mistake.

The sooner we accept the imperfect nature of healthcare and learn from our mistakes, the quicker patients and providers might forgive each other and themselves, and the better we can all recover from the physical, emotional, and financial wounds these errors inflict. By recognizing that we are all in this together, we can do a better job keeping patients and those who care for them safe from unnecessary harm.

I wrote this book because I am convinced public engagement through the creation of community coalitions can accelerate improvement in patient safety across the United States. *Your Patient Safety Survival Guide* presents a blueprint that can be adapted to meet the needs and interests of various hospitals and communities. Regardless of one's interest in forming a coalition, this book offers information and action plans to help safeguard individual patients and healthcare providers. It draws on personal experiences, although names of real people and organizations have been disguised unless the incidents were previously publicized.

CHAPTER 1

Help Me, Heal Me, Don't Harm Me
How Healthcare Frequently Injures Patients

There is no single medical intervention that will ever save as many lives as patient safety improvement. There is so much harm going on.[1]

—Donald Berwick, MD, Institute for Healthcare Improvement

The task is . . . not so much to see what no one has yet seen; but to think what nobody has yet thought, about that which everybody sees.[2]

—Erwin Schrödinger (1847–1961)

THE MAGNITUDE OF THE PATIENT SAFETY CRISIS

If you aren't concerned about being treated (or working) in a hospital, you should be. Keeping people safe during the delivery of healthcare is one of the greatest challenges facing modern medicine. In spite of the best intentions and Herculean efforts of millions of American doctors, nurses, pharmacists, allied health professionals, and patient safety advocates, at least 440,000 patients die needless deaths in US hospitals each year.[3]

For those who don't relate well to dry statistics, this means that medical errors are now the third leading cause of death in the United States—far ahead of deaths due to auto accidents, diabetes, and everything else except cancer and heart disease.[4] As one healthcare leader put it, these numbers mean "hospitals are killing off the equivalent of the entire population of Atlanta one year, Miami the next, then moving to Oakland, and on and on."[5] The equivalent of four Vietnam Memorials would need to be built each year to capture the names of US hospital patients who die as a result of hospital-induced harm.

We would consider any other industry that inflicted harm on so many of its customers to be catastrophically unsafe. The reality is any business with such a track record would be shut down or boycotted. But healthcare confers innumerable benefits, such that it is deemed essential to life. Thus, boycotting hospitals and locking their doors are not viable options, and we must bear the mistakes and associated costs until we make healthcare safer.

An initial estimate of the financial impact of the patient safety crisis indicated it totaled around $5 billion annually, about one-quarter of which involves out-of-pocket expenses.[6] However, that figure is outdated and probably always represented a gross underestimate of the true cost of medical mistakes. A more recent analysis, which included a greater number of studies and more comprehensive data-capturing methods, indicated that the excess cost related to hospital-acquired infections alone—just one of many patient safety problems—would be between $28 billion and $45 billion annually in 2007 dollars.[7] In today's dollars, this would equate to between $32 and $52 billion annually. And when the indirect costs for lost workdays and short-term disability claims are accounted for, the total outlay for healthcare-associated infections may be as high as $1 trillion annually.[8]

As astounding as these figures are, they represent conservative estimates—not exaggerated claims—and they do not tell the whole story. Over the past five years or so, most US hospitals have implemented electronic health record systems. These systems have made it possible to more accurately determine how often healthcare causes harm to patients. Information extracted directly from patients' hospital records indicates that the problem is ten times higher than previous estimates: one out of every three hospital patients is inappropriately harmed during the process of receiving care.[9]

Rates of harm are incomplete, whether they are generated from voluntary reports or from information extracted from electronic medical records. First, both methods tend to overlook errors of omission and diagnostic errors that only become evident in the days, weeks, and months after patients leave the hospital. Research indicates that one in five patients will experience an adverse event after being discharged from the hospital—and many of these will represent what should have been preventable return visits to an emergency department or hospital readmissions.[10] Second, neither method tallies the harm that occurs as a result of mistakes made in freestanding surgical centers, nursing homes, or outpatient clinics. Finally, the majority of American physicians acknowledge that they sometimes choose not to report serious medical errors of which they have firsthand knowledge,[11] and some alter records or leave them incomplete to obfuscate the evidence of harm.[12]

Healthcare providers may perpetuate harm; however, sometimes they also are secondary victims of patient tragedies. Among physicians who have been involved in a serious safety event, up to two-thirds report that the experience undermined their job confidence and satisfaction.[13] Many providers experience lingering anxiety, guilt, and fear—emotional devastation that causes some to perform suboptimally or leave the field altogether. Although medical mishaps can shake providers to their core, we do a poor job of alleviating their trauma or the related problems of burnout and on-the-job physical injuries. Hospitals are one of the most hazardous places to work, with an employee injury rate that is nearly twice as high as all private industries combined. "It is more hazardous to work in a hospital than to work in construction or manufacturing."[14] None of this type of hospital-related suffering is considered when assessing the magnitude or cost of the patient safety crisis.

Whatever the ultimate magnitude of healthcare-induced harm, there is universal agreement that it is far too great.[15] Before there can be any real hope of curtailing this epidemic, more providers and consumers of healthcare must take charge.

WHAT A PATIENT SAFETY EVENT LOOKS LIKE

To be clear, we are not talking about people dying from the illnesses that caused them to seek treatment in the first place. We are also not talking about complications that result from procedures where known risks are perceived as worthwhile compared to the likely outcome if the procedure is not performed. *Patient safety events* refer to wrongful events of healthcare-induced harm and death. These events are not due to breakdowns in complex medical decision making or the lack of access to care. Most often, patient safety events involve basic human and system error. "None of us is ever very far from a terrible medical mistake."[16] So, what does a terrible medical mistake or a patient safety event look like?

It is the teenager whose skin and organs have been ravaged and permanently deformed by a superbug infection that he picked up in the hospital because people neglected to wash their hands.

It is the mother-to-be who had the wrong embryo transplanted into her womb because the in vitro clinic didn't use the universally approved preoperative checklist, leaving the mother to cope with a court order to share custody of the child with a complete stranger—the man whose sperm was used to create the embryo that grew to be her baby.

It is the newborn whose heart stops after receiving a medication dose that was calculated for an adult because an overworked pharmacist made a mistake and a nurse did not double-check the order before injecting the drug into the baby's IV.

Every single day, these errors kill one thousand hospital patients and cause serious harm to another ten thousand to twenty thousand. Nobody is immune—not doctors, nurses, or hospital CEOs. It happens to newborn babies, pregnant mothers, and the elderly. It has happened to me, and it could happen to you.

THE UNDERREPORTED DISASTER AND ITS UNTAPPED RESOURCE

In an average week—week, not year—more patients will die from the care they receive in US hospitals than the total number of people who died in natural disasters between 2005 and 2015, including Hurricane Katrina and the massive earthquakes in Nepal. Among the nine deadliest natural disasters since 1900, only the great China Flood of 1931 had a death toll that surpasses the weekly rate of preventable death in American hospitals. While hurricanes, tsunamis, earthquakes, and other natural disasters make national news and receive round-the-clock coverage, the patient safety death toll climbs week after week with scant media attention or public awareness.

Along with the press coverage of natural disasters comes thousands of people who freely give their time, talent, and resources to help stabilize the situation and heal the afflicted. If the American public understood the magnitude of the patient safety crisis and had a clear idea of how they could make hospitals safer, they would offer a helping hand. But here's the rub: even if the public stepped up to help, healthcare workers aren't prepared to accept their help. That is why I decided to write this book—to help prepare patients to act as genuine partners in safe care while also encouraging providers to embrace this help.

If the best clinicians, scientists, regulators, and policymakers working in tandem haven't been able to solve this problem, why should anyone expect the solution to depend on getting the public involved? After all, we are talking about a vexing problem that occurs during the course of complex clinical care within an industry that operates at a rapid pace, under the toll of extensive regulation, and in the midst of a constantly changing knowledge base. So, you might wonder, why complicate the problem by getting the public involved?

The truth is that the public cannot solve the patient safety crisis on its own any more than hospitals can. Radically improving patient safety will require meaningful collaboration—a true partnership—among providers and patients and between hospitals and the communities they serve. Such collaboration must be the norm; it must not remain a lofty ideal or the exception to the rule. And waiting until patients are hospitalized, or about to be hospitalized, to prepare them for their roles and responsibilities for safe care amounts to too little too late.

THE EVOLUTION OF PATIENT SAFETY TRAINING, 1900–2000

For over one hundred years, beginning in the early 1900s and long before the term "patient safety" ever came into vogue, surgeons and anesthesiologists routinely learned from patient safety events. They participated in what they called morbidity and mortality, or M&M, conferences. These regularly scheduled hospital-based conferences were considered a place where physicians could freely discuss unexpectedly bad outcomes with trusted colleagues. Eventually, the Accreditation Council for Graduate Medical Education and other physician residency programs mandated that M&M conferences become part of physician training. As these conferences became a more integral part of physician training, M&M cases were often selected for presentation based on their instructive value for residents rather than the ability to improve an understanding of medical mistakes.

Besides M&M conferences no longer being a dependable source of patient safety education per se, medicine has been slow to incorporate the field's accumulating knowledge into its textbooks and medical school curricula.[17] With the exponential growth of medical science, it has been challenging to fit the newly emerging body of patient safety knowledge into established clinical courses. While there are massive efforts underway to strengthen patient safety education in medical schools and to improve continuing education standards for physicians, the reality is that physician sensitivity to the topic of patient safety is not yet universally viewed as an essential aspect of physician selection, training, or evaluation.[18]

By default, a lot of patient safety education has been relegated to on-the-job training. Once physicians graduate and enter the workforce, it is not necessarily easy for them to learn about the science and practice of patient safety. With pressing needs to remain current on rapidly evolving topics of clinical care, most physicians choose to travel to conferences related to their clinical specialties rather than on patient safety. So, in-house patient safety training is of paramount importance. Yet many hospitals routinely exempt physicians from such training. A stated reason has been that because most of their physicians function as independent practitioners rather than hospital employees, hospital administrators cannot require them to participate in hospital training. Exempting physicians is unfortunate because physicians are regarded as team leaders.

With physicians at the top of the medical hierarchy, how they are educated about patient safety has a major influence over what gets incorporated into academic training programs for nurses, pharmacists, and allied health professionals. When doctors are not prepared to support hospital safety initiatives, nurses and other staff will not take them seriously, or at least they won't for long.

During the course of a consulting engagement with a large and highly respected urban hospital, physicians refused to join in-house safety training sessions alongside nurses and other staff members. Whatever length of time was necessary to cover the topic with employees, the physicians felt they could learn the material faster. My colleagues and I did not necessarily agree; in fact, some of us strongly believed in the value of cross-disciplinary training. Nonetheless, we seized an opportunity to arrange for a notable safety expert to provide a brief, free, and physician-only seminar on patient safety at the hospital. The seminar was specifically designed for physicians. In spite of the recruiting efforts by the hospital's department that oversaw safety and quality work, only a handful of doctors showed up for the training. Just like parenting programs that seem to attract the most competent parents rather than those most in need of guidance, the physicians who attended the seminar were already recognized as notable in-house patient safety champions.

BIRTH OF THE PATIENT SAFETY MOVEMENT, 1995–2005

For centuries, the magnitude of preventable deaths was underappreciated and underreported. This changed in an "instant" with the publication of the now legendary report by the National Academies of Science's Institute of Medicine, aptly titled *To Err Is Human*.[19] Release of this report marked a turning point in medical history. It was the first time that the field of medicine disclosed to the public the extent to which hospital patients are needlessly harmed in the process of receiving care and the industry's lack of a systematic approach to prevent such harm.[20]

The considerable press associated with the release of the report is commonly marked as the start of the patient safety movement. Dr. Lucian Leape, the physician who conducted one of the two large-scale studies on which *To Err Is Human* was based and who is now recognized as the father of the academic field of patient safety, has noted that crucial events preceded the media frenzy over the report. In 1995, for example, a number of egregious patient safety events made front-page news; the attorney for the American Medical Association "prodded" the organization to form a group of stakeholders to promote patient safety; and the head of the Veteran's Administration decided to make safety a system priority.[21] But the media's focus on the report and the federal government's response to it set other critical actions in motion.

Most significantly, the release of *To Err Is Human* removed the medical profession's own blinders to the magnitude of preventable hospital deaths. Before the report was released, preventable fatalities simply had not been regularly tallied or publicized. Thus, individual doctors and nurses had no way of knowing how the isolated errors that they or their colleagues witnessed or experienced added up on a hospital, community, or national scale. Over the last fifteen years, however, the field of patient safety has been advancing its knowledge of healthcare-induced harm and how to prevent it. But far too many healthcare professionals and patients still know far too little about how they contribute to the problem or what they can do to solve it.

In spite of the initial and strong backlash from some quarters suggesting that *To Err Is Human* overestimated the magnitude of the problem (a criticism that with the benefit of hindsight was clearly proved wrong), the federal government set a national goal of reducing the number of preventable healthcare-induced deaths by 50 percent between 2000 and 2005. In 2001, Congress appropriated $50 million for patient safety research. As a result, for the first time in modern medicine studying patient safety became a legitimate pursuit, and journals were created for the purpose of establishing repositories of knowledge about patient safety.

Existing and newly formed patient safety-oriented organizations began buzzing with passionate focus and activity directed toward improving patient outcomes, including the US Agency for Healthcare Research and Quality and the Joint Commission (the largest hospital and healthcare accrediting agency in the United States), as well as major nonprofit organizations such as the Institute for Healthcare Improvement and National Patient Safety Forum—all of which continue to play a vital role in advancing safe patient care.

For somewhat different reasons, leaders of Fortune 500 companies and other large public and private purchasers of healthcare benefits weighed in on *To Err Is Human*. They were distraught over paying for healthcare coverage for their employees when such coverage might actually lead to harm. It was particularly concerning to them that they had no way to determine which hospitals or healthcare plans were more likely to be associated with bad outcomes for their employees and high costs to their businesses. By the end of 2000, these leaders coalesced to form what is known as The Leapfrog Group.

To this day, The Leapfrog Group is a powerful consumer-oriented consortium of businesses with a mission to trigger giant leaps forward in healthcare safety and quality. Leapfrog continues to press the envelope with respect to hospital transparency and public reporting of patient safety and quality metrics, making it easier for businesses and individuals to be more informed when choosing their healthcare providers. As summed up by Leapfrog's president and CEO, Leah Binder (who repeatedly has been listed among the top fifty professionals who positively impact healthcare), "I run an organization . . . with a membership of highly impatient business leaders fed up with problems of injuries, accidents, and errors in hospitals."[22]

And so, within months of *To Err Is Human* going public, the patient safety movement was born.

SAFETY CULTURE WORK IN AMERICAN HOSPITALS, 2005–2010

Five years into the movement, American hospitals had invested a great amount of effort and capital to improve patient safety. Nearly every healthcare worker, regardless of his or her professional background, had become aware of the patient safety crisis. By 2005, nobody doubted that the patient safety crisis was every bit as real as first suggested by *To Err Is Human*. The walls of silence and denial had come crumbling down. But by 2005, it was also clear that healthcare had not achieved—or even come close to achieving—its goal of reducing preventable deaths by 50 percent on a national level. In fact, there was no evidence of widespread improvement. There simply had been no downshift in the magnitude of the crisis.[23] While leaders of the movement were stressed by the lack of obvious progress, they had laid important groundwork for future success.

When I joined the field in 2007, hospital safety efforts were intense and intensifying. Healthcare leaders had already turned to nuclear power engineers and aviation psychologists for help because these industries experienced fewer than one in a million safety disasters. Healthcare wanted to be like commercial aviation and nuclear power—

industries that had figured out how to minimize safety disasters while maintaining high-volume, high-risk operations. *High reliability organizations*, or HROs, are business entities that are reliably safe despite their inherently high-risk, high-volume endeavors. Drawing on the lessons learned by safety experts working with HRO companies, healthcare policymakers, leaders, and consultants agreed on the components that were essential to building a culture of safety in hospitals.

Dominant consultancy organizations marketed fundamental HRO concepts to hospitals around the country. First and foremost, they considered (and still consider) it essential that hospital leaders view safety as a core value. Adopting *safety as a core value* means that safety is a precondition for the delivery of clinical care and that safety cannot be compromised to the service of productivity or other potentially competing priorities. As a natural extension of holding safety as a core value, hospitals followed a three-step process of setting clear expectations for safe behavior, educating staff about such behavioral expectations, and building accountability around adherence to established expectations.[24] To model themselves after high-risk industries with stellar safety records, hospitals also recognized the need to develop programs to investigate serious safety events for the purpose of finding and fixing their root causes. The strongest programs began sharing the lessons they learned about errors and serious mishaps with employees throughout their hospitals and broader healthcare systems. Some even started to post stories of patient safety events that had transpired in their facilities on websites for the public to see.

Between 2005 and 2010, hospital-based safety culture programs proliferated, and it wasn't long before almost every hospital worker was familiar with the term *safety culture* and at least a few HRO concepts. However, by 2010, American hospitals still had not come close to achieving HRO status. While safety culture work had fostered incredibly important breakthroughs in narrowly defined clinical issues, such as ways to eliminate infections associated with specific medical procedures, the country's overall rate of preventable hospital deaths had not declined. In spite of astounding dedication by hospital leaders around the country, ten years into the movement patient safety leaders were disheartened to report that—yet again—there was no sign of general improvement.[25]

Healthcare is distinctly different from industries that have achieved HRO status. Healthcare centers on people, and people are dynamic beings whose behavior cannot be controlled to the same degree as equipment (airplanes), physical structures (power plants), or materials (chemicals). While safety culture work wasn't producing the level of results that healthcare was looking for on a national level, the industry thought (and many proclaimed) that standardizing clinical operations through the use of technology could lead to radical improvements in patient safety. Then along came the Health Information Technology for Economic and Clinical Health (HITECH) Act of 2009.

HEALTH INFORMATION TECHNOLOGY HYPE AND HOPE, 2009–2013

The HITECH Act refers to federal legislation that included $19.2 billion to stimulate a digital revolution in the healthcare industry by promoting rapid adoption of electronic health records in hospitals and clinics across the nation. Through Medicaid and Medicare resources, the federal government offered financial incentives for hospitals and medical practices that were early adopters of electronic health records and levied financial penalties for those who did not make measurable progress by specific target dates.

The HITECH legislation and its associated stimulus funding and policies infused the patient safety movement with a dose of hope; and, once again, hospitals responded in a commendable fashion. Even in spite of trepidations about the logistics and costs of implementing electronic health record systems, hospitals (and outpatient clinics) rapidly began implementing electronic health records in ways that had a meaningful impact on patient care. Whereas only 12 percent of acute care hospitals had even a basic electronic health record system in place in 2008, as of May 2014, 94 percent had a system in place that met federal certification requirements.[26]

This digital revolution contributed to seismic improvements in the way health information was captured, stored, and retrieved from patient records. Nonetheless, the use of electronic health records did not lessen the overall magnitude of the patient safety crisis.[27] In fact, it quickly became apparent that these systems created new opportunities for error while controlling for known sources of error. Furthermore, in the rush to implement these systems, too little attention was paid to the human side of safety, including the human interface with technology.[28]

From 2010 to 2013, I served as one of the country's five regional leaders for the HITECH consortium of community colleges that was charged with developing and implementing new programs to prepare a workforce to support the use of electronic health records. To my dismay, none of my four counterparts had any notable expertise in patient safety. Likewise, none of the program directors or managers of the community colleges within my thirteen-state HITECH region did either. I was concerned about the fact that the HITECH workforce initiative was flooding the market with newly minted electronic health record professionals with minimal training on patient safety. And I thought it would be irresponsible to not use some portion of the $16 million HITECH grant I was directing to deliver patient safety education to those who were designing and overseeing electronic health record training and educational programs.

Fortunately, HITECH grant officers allowed a portion of the federal funding to be used to host a national conference on the topic of patient safety in the digital era. Conference attendees were impressed with the dynamic keynote talks delivered by Leah Binder (Leapfrog president and CEO) and David Classen, MD (renowned health information technology innovator). But few, if any, conference participants consequently strengthened the patient safety component of their programs. Like medical schools, it seemed community colleges were leaving much of the necessary education about patient safety to on-the-job training.

In spite of past and current disappointments and limitations of electronic health record systems and the ways in which they are (and are not) used, they are here to stay. As eloquently explained in *The Digital Doctor* by physician Robert Wachter, one of the field's champions and examiners of reform, this is a good thing.[29] While working with numerous hospitals during their transitions from paper to digital systems, I never encountered a professional who did not eventually—if not immediately—see the value of electronic health record systems.

TEMPORARY DISILLUSIONMENT, 2013–2015

By 2013, the Joint Commission's president and chief executive officer and its executive vice president publicly admitted defeat in their effort to stem the tide of patient safety events. They lamented that in the wake of safety culture work and the adoption of electronic health record systems, hospitals were suffering from project fatigue. They noted that no hospital had managed to successfully adapt the science of safety to the business of healthcare. They declared the performance of American hospitals to be predictably unreliable and unsafe and that no amount of regulation could make them safe.[30] It is an extraordinary day when leaders of the most significant healthcare regulatory body assert that more regulation will not solve the problem at hand. So it is not shocking that by 2013, there was blog chatter about the patient safety movement flickering out.[31]

To make matters worse, the following year, the patient safety movement was rocked by its first scandal. The scandal centered on Dr. Charles Denham, the man who had been a darling of the movement, with connections to people in high places from Hollywood to the White House; the man who produced a slick video about the importance of patient safety that his consulting firm provided free of charge to hospitals around the country; the man who, after suddenly appearing on the scene from left field, managed to position himself as a board member or chair of several major patient safety organizations and as the editor of the *Journal of Patient Safety*. In 2014, it was discovered that Denham was under federal investigation for having accepted over $11 million from CareFusion, a company that manufactured safety-related products, apparently to infiltrate the field and use his position of authority to lobby for policies that directly advantaged CareFusion. The government settled the case with a $40 million payment by CareFusion and a $1 million payment by Denham. The settlement precludes the public from ever knowing details of the case. Denham never admitted to the charges, but he did dupe a lot of people.

For example, while serving as a cochair of the National Patient Safety Forum, which vetted safety-related products, Denham successfully lobbied the organization to unjustly and unfairly recommend a specific product for preventing bloodstream infections—a product that only CareFusion produced. Denham's path to becoming editor of the *Journal of Patient Safety* turned out to involve undue pressure and unprecedented actions that are inconsistent with academic standards. Under his editorial watch, Denham authored and published papers in the journal that had clear and undisclosed conflicts of interest.

Until the Denham scandal broke, the field of patient safety had rested on its laurels, assuming that everyone was a do-gooder with pure intentions. With hindsight, it was painfully obvious that there were plenty of red flags about Denham's motives, as well as his sudden rise to prominence and tendency to lavish compliments and support toward the movement's prominent projects and people.[32, 33] The Denham scandal marked the end of innocence for the movement. Like other areas of the healthcare industry, the patient safety movement had to come to terms with the reality that billions of dollars rest on which policies, practices, and products flourish and which ones die.

A PARADIGM SHIFT—ZEROING IN FOR SUCCESS

In 2010, my work began focusing primarily on helping industrial and manufacturing companies improve the safety culture in their organizations; however, I kept watching what was happening in healthcare—something that was possible, in part, because Leah Binder and David Classen, along with other colleagues of his, graciously invited me to attend annual conferences hosted by The Leapfrog Group and Pascal Metrics. Watching things unfold, it occurred to me that, as I described in an article published in *Society*, a fundamental change in our nation's approach to and assumptions about patient safety seems to be in order.[34] The premise of that article and this book is the same: a paradigm shift is necessary, and it must center on engaging patients for the purpose of collaborating with healthcare providers to eliminate a small but powerful subset of patient safety's most frequently recurring problems. A decidedly narrow focus that simultaneously engages those who receive and deliver healthcare would finally place within reach the national goal of reducing hospital-induced harm by 50 percent within a five-year period—the goal that was set in 2000 and that healthcare has never come close to achieving.

There are sound reasons to narrow the focus of hospital safety programs. With zeal for improvement, hospital and industry leaders have been designing and championing safety programs that aim to tackle a multitude of issues simultaneously. They tend to blur the distinction between the broad area of quality and its narrower subset of patient safety. Although safe care represents one way of measuring overall quality of care, there are differences between safety and quality. Quality improvements have more to do with the selection and timing of clinical interventions (what and when care gets delivered) while safety efforts have more to do with the manner in which people go about the business of delivering care (how care gets delivered).

Quality-related work covers an innumerable array of complex topics and potential solutions that must be examined across a wide range of patient populations, practice settings, and clinician groups. Establishing what constitutes high-quality or evidence-based medicine is generally initiated, validated, and incorporated into the delivery system through the efforts of a select subset of healthcare professionals with ties to universities and academic medical centers. In contrast, advances in safe care generally pertain to rules, practices, and systems for getting all healthcare workers to consistently or habitually perform a small number of relatively straightforward behaviors, such as washing hands before entering and after exiting patient rooms. While some quality initiatives eventually inform safe practice, it is helpful to appreciate and bracket their unique contributions.

Laudable as comprehensive quality/safety efforts are for advancing medical science, as organization-wide programs or initiatives designed to improve day-to-day safety at the bedside, they set healthcare workers up for failure, disappointment, and disillusion. Greater return on investment can be realized by focusing on getting providers en masse to exhibit excellent performance around a defined and manageable set of safety habits. Because safety depends on patients being part of the solution, it is all the more important to focus on habits they too can recognize, request, and/or use. Yet a recent survey indicated that half of the American population is still unfamiliar with the term patient safety, although a growing number are concerned with medical mistakes—obviously not having connected the two.[35]

Psychologists who specialize in behavior change know that people are capable of addressing only one or two new behavioral habits or routines at a time. The same holds true for establishing organizational habits.

A TRIFECTA OF PREVALENT, PREDICTABLE, AND PREVENTABLE SAFETY PROBLEMS

In the fifteen years since the hospital safety crisis was publicly exposed, the field of patient safety has identified specific strategies that have the capacity to eliminate the vast majority of hospital deaths due to (1) healthcare-associated infections, (2) off-the-mark procedures,[36] and (3) medication administration errors. The safety strategies to prevent these three event types involve simple, quick, and practically cost-free actions, such as the use of proper handwashing, checklists, and double checks. As a group, these event types comprise the majority of all preventable deaths that occur in US hospitals, representing a safety trifecta of sorts.[37]

Not only does this trifecta of safety events represent the most prevalent, predictable, and preventable types of patient harm with which hospitals must cope, they also happen to constitute exactly the sort of problems that public health interventions are capable of successfully addressing. These event types clearly represent the field's low-hanging fruit. The associated safety habits involve behaviors that healthcare workers must use regardless of the facility, so a unified public health approach has the added advantage of setting consistent expectations for physicians and staff who change jobs or work in multiple locations.

Therefore, narrowing and coordinating the focus of institutional efforts and public engagement around hospital safety's current trifecta, or any one of its component issues, would finally place within reach the national goal of drastically cutting the rate of harm over a period of a few years. But the field must be willing to do less to achieve more, and to accommodate some shifts in power from those who deliver care to those who receive it.

OUR BEST HOPE FOR SUCCESS

No matter how sophisticated the science of medicine or clinical care delivery systems become, it is an inescapable reality that ensuring patient safety is often a function of forming and sustaining simple safety habits among the millions of nurses, physicians, pharmacists, therapists, support staff, and others who affect the lives of patients every day. The breadth and volume of people who must exhibit safety habits begs for a unified, straightforward, and manageable approach. The work before us calls for a paradigm that is comprehensible to everyone regardless of rank or role and that unifies efforts of hospitals, public health, and society overall.

To the extent they are capable, providers and consumers of healthcare need to know and exercise their roles and responsibilities for eliminating healthcare's current trifecta of safety events. Building accountability around the safety habits that can eliminate these recurring serious safety events depends on creating a greater sense that providers are accountable to their patients while also preparing patients to speak up when they observe lapses in their healthcare.

Having held leadership positions in hospitals, conducted public health research, and chaired a community-based coalition, I am confident that the field of patient safety can make a giant leap forward by expanding the safety culture model to be consistent with a more comprehensive public health framework.

CHAPTER 2

What Seems Too Simple to Matter Could Save Your Life

Leverage the Power of Safety Habits

Incompetent people are, at most, 1% of the problem. The other 99% are good people trying to do a good job who make very simple mistakes and it's the processes that set them up to make these mistakes.[1]

—Lucien Leape, MD, Harvard School of Public Health

Excellence is an art won by training and habituation. We do not act rightly because we have virtue or excellence, but we rather have those because we have acted rightly. We are what we repeatedly do. Excellence, then, is not an act but a habit.

—Aristotle, Greek philosopher (384 BC–322 BC)

FIRST THINGS FIRST

We have a natural desire to fix everything all at once because any safety mishap that harms a patient is one too many; the life of every patient matters. Indeed, the field of patient safety must not lose sight of the full array of patient safety problems. And yet, the most efficient way to accelerate sweeping improvement is to focus on problems that affect large numbers of people and can also be solved with simple solutions. That is why it makes sense to concentrate the movement's efforts on the trifecta of infections, procedural mistakes, and medication administration errors. Doing so can help us transform the complex problem of patient safety into manageable pieces that can be tackled systematically.

To understand the logic and value of purposefully focusing and simplifying patient safety efforts, it helps to suspend any sense of urgency to reduce *all* instances of harm for the sake of eradicating *specific* instances of harm. For a moment, take these things, which will be borne out in the coming chapters, on faith:

- Healthcare has identified specific safety behaviors that can, when used consistently, eliminate or radically reduce harm associated with the most prevalent, predictable, and preventable types of patient safety problems—a trifecta of safety events.
- The safety habits that can effectively prevent healthcare's current trifecta of safety events are simple, take about two and a half minutes or less to complete, and are essentially cost-free.
- Virtually every healthcare worker needs to be proficient in using the safety habits for preventing the field's current trifecta of patient safety events.

Think about patient safety events occurring along a continuum, from those solutions that are relatively straightforward to those solutions that are extremely complex and complicated. The current trifecta anchors the easy end of the patient safety continuum.

How so? First, we already know what needs to be done to prevent healthcare-associated infections, off-the-mark procedures, and most medication administration errors. Second, the nature of the solutions to these problems involves specific behavioral actions—not complex or clinical procedures. Third, the requisite behavioral actions amount to safety habits that every healthcare professional must develop. Fourth, most patients (or their lay caregivers) can be taught to observe whether the requisite safety habits are used during clinical encounters. Finally, a proven strategy already exists for raising public awareness and mobilizing action to coordinate change around observable events and scripted actions (see chapter 6).

This analysis suggests that the greatest barrier to improving performance around some of patient safety's most common problems is not a matter of medical science. It is a matter of getting people to do what they know is important, and this requires the aid of behavioral science. Because of the volume of providers and patients who must become engaged in the process, making a dent in the patient safety crisis will also require the aid of public health practitioners, as well as individuals, groups, and organizations that do not have a formal connection to healthcare.

When thinking about patient safety events along this continuum of challenging problems, it becomes obvious which of the field's problems are ready to scale up for widespread success. For the reasons just described, it seems clear that each of the current trifecta events is ready for prime time. Preventing patient falls and pressure ulcers (bedsores from lying in one position for too long) may be next in line. On the one hand, patient falls and pressure ulcers are like the trifecta events in that they are highly prevalent and predictable problems whose prevention strategies primarily involve behavioral actions that must be consistently followed. On the other hand, they are unlike the trifecta events in that the preventative safety habits are required only for a subset of at-risk patients. Some hospital units already have had success reducing patient falls and pressure ulcers; however, because these event types are not as universally relevant to all patients and providers, it makes reasonable sense to tackle them after healthcare has experienced success in building the necessary organizational and community architecture to address patient safety issues that affect everyone.

The opposite end of the continuum is anchored by thorny problems, which include misdiagnosis and delays in diagnosis. Preventing diagnostic errors may be patient safety's most challenging problem. In fact, solutions for this class of events are likely to be so numerous and idiosyncratic, relative to the type of condition and/or diagnostic tests and/or facilities involved. Because solutions are also likely to be specialty-specific, tackling diagnostic errors is arguably a matter that is more suitable to the broader field of quality improvement around clinical issues rather than the subdomain of patient safety. Healthcare will grapple with complex issues like the elimination of diagnostic errors for a long time to come, if not indefinitely. However, the existence of endlessly challenging quality and safety issues must not obscure the benefit of tackling other distinct safety issues with immediate and co-ordinated decisiveness.

NO BAD APPLES

Given that low-cost or no-cost solutions already exist for healthcare's current trifecta, why do they persist as a major problem in virtually every hospital? Why do even the best physicians and nurses who have been trained to use essential safety habits disregard them, and why does healthcare tolerate their suboptimal performance? The truth is, getting people to consistently use known error-prevention strategies isn't as easy as one might think.

Take the case of healthcare-associated infections that harm millions of lives and cost billions of dollars each year. Since 2001, The Leapfrog Group has been surveying hospitals about their hand-hygiene policies to see if they expect providers to adhere to standards that are known to prevent patients from picking up infections during the course of a hospital visit. According to Leapfrog's CEO, Leah Binder, a patient's risk of dying is two to four times lower if they receive care in a hospital that meets Leapfrog standards. If most hospitals followed the basic infection-prevention practices tracked by the Leapfrog Hospital Survey, fifty-seven thousand lives and $12 billion could be saved each year. Yet as of 2012, Leapfrog reported that, among the hospitals that agreed to be voluntarily surveyed and have their results publicly reported, only 62 percent even had hygiene policies in place.[2] Fortunately, by 2013, the figure had risen by fifteen percentage points.[3]

That a sizable portion of reporting hospitals still doesn't have a handwashing policy in place is disconcerting. In defense of hospitals, let's assume they are concerned about implementing policies they cannot enforce. To be compliant with evidence-based handwashing standards, providers must wash their hands every time they enter and exit a patient's room. Over the course of an average day, this alone could easily amount to as many as forty instances of handwashing for a typical outpatient physician, sometimes more and sometimes less for hospital physicians and staff. Even among individuals who are highly motivated to comply with best practice standards, the hustle and bustle of the dynamic hospital setting will, at times, interfere with their resolve.

Another challenge to turning essential safety behaviors into reliable habits is this: it is virtually impossible for healthcare providers to see a link between any one of their own safety lapses and an instance of direct harm to one of their patients. Sometimes this happens because the error has no discernable effect; other times it is because the error's effect does not become apparent until later. As a result, we often maintain nonoptimal behavioral patterns with no real feedback to spur behavior change.

Take a classic example of a child and a hot stove. The child has been told not to touch the hot stove because bad things will happen. It will hurt, he will get burned, and he may have to go to the hospital. So, for a long time, the child never touches the stove. One day, though, his bouncy ball lands on the counter, precariously perched on the edge of the hot stove. To retrieve the ball, he either needs to wait for his mother to stop what she is doing and help him or put his hand dangerously close to the hot burner to retrieve it himself. He decides to take a risk. He reaches up to the stove, puts his hand near the burner, and gets burned.

In this scenario, a risk was taken and a sufficiently unpleasant negative consequence occurred immediately. A clear connection was made between the child's behavior and the negative consequence. You can bet that child will not be taking that risk again anytime soon. Imagine, though, if the same scenario occurred but the child placed his hand just far enough from the burner that he did not get burned. His workaround would have been successful. Not only would his risky behavior not have been punished, it would actually have been rewarded. So the child would never know how close he had come to being seriously hurt and would be more likely to take the same risk again.

It is simply unfair (and unhelpful) to blame providers for comparable breakdowns in the care-delivery process. They are not "bad apples"; they are dedicated people who have been set up for failure. Errors, especially recurring minor errors, point to system failures. We cannot overcome the human propensity for error through sheer willpower, so it is unrealistic to expect providers to consistently do the right thing simply because they possess the knowledge that the given behavior is important. Perhaps it is no wonder that so many hospitals have avoided creating handwashing policies or fail to enforce them.

So, what can be done to create the possibility for hospitals to expect and build accountability around essential safety behaviors—the behaviors that take place every day and often behind pulled curtains or closed doors?

GETTING PATIENTS IN THE GAME

One solution is to create a greater sense that providers are accountable to the patients they serve while also preparing patients to speak up when they observe lapses among their healthcare providers' safety habits. Now that dangerous infections like Methicillin-resistant Staphylococcus aureus (MRSA, pronounced mersa) are spreading beyond hospital walls and into outpatient settings, as well as the broader community (schools, daycare centers, and gyms),[4] the public has good reason to be mindful of whether people walking in and out of patient rooms wash their hands. In fact, there may be no other patient safety issue that stands to gain from urgent and concerted efforts to engage the public.

If patients truly understood the importance of proper hand hygiene, they would be more vigilant about whether or not it happened in their presence. What is needed is a way to raise public awareness, motivate civic action, and offer patients, lay caregivers, and those who visit them in the hospital manageable steps for ensuring consistent handwashing. As you will see in coming chapters, the same holds true for off-the-mark procedures and medication administration errors. That is, the public needs to understand the simple safety habits that can protect them from harm and how to make sure they are used during the care that they and their loved ones receive.

ANOTHER SLICE OF CHEESE, PLEASE!

In the 1990s, psychologist James Reason introduced a model that he originally intended to be used for academic purposes by fellow cognitive psychologists who studied large-scale disasters like airplane crashes and nuclear power plant meltdowns.[5] This model, which he dubbed the *Swiss Cheese Model*, turned out to be exceptionally useful for understanding how workplace conditions affect on-the-job performance. It quickly became and continues to be the dominant framework for guiding the development of safety programs across a wide range of high-risk industries, including healthcare.

The Swiss Cheese Model recognizes that human error is unavoidably common. People will make mistakes—it is human nature, a given reality, and a fact of life that we must accept. According to the model, however, we can build safety nets to prevent common and potentially serious mistakes from happening. That is, human error cannot be totally eliminated, but human error can be caught, stopped, or prevented before it leads to major mishaps or disastrous events.

To understand the Swiss Cheese Model, look at the graphic below and think of each slice as being a protective barrier. Using the Swiss cheese analogy, a straw (error) could pass all the way through a stack of slices of Swiss cheese (protective barriers) only if all the holes (barrier imperfections, weaknesses, and vulnerabilities) happened to be perfectly aligned—as represented by the arrow. Tragedy strikes—patients are harmed—only when the straw (error) manages to get all the way through the cheese (when all protective barriers fail). Reason's model recognizes the need for *barriers in depth*, meaning that because any one barrier is imperfect, as represented by the holes in the Swiss cheese, generally the more protective barriers we put in place, the safer the system. For high-risk undertakings, barriers in depth are essential for a condition of safety to prevail.

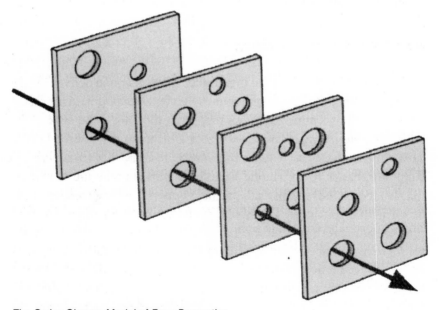

The Swiss Cheese Model of Error Prevention.
Source: Gretchen LeFever Watson.

The Swiss Cheese Model also asserts that most accidents represent system-level breakdowns, not malicious acts by bad people. It turns the "bad apple" mentality on its head. Recognizing that doctors and nurses do not set out to hurt their patients, the question to ask when a mistake occurs is: What led the person involved to believe that what he or she did was the right action at that time? In healthcare, the answer is too often that nobody was there to remind well-intentioned caregivers to do the right thing. In other words, the necessary slice of cheese is missing at precisely the time and place that it was needed most.

Patients will often be the last people to have the chance to remind healthcare workers to use common safety behaviors, and patients have the most at stake when safety precautions are disregarded. This is why we urgently need to equip patients for their vital role in safety. The stakes are too high to continue to work without patients serving as genuine partners in safe care. Using the Swiss cheese analogy, patients and their lay caregivers need to act as a final protective barrier (a slice of Swiss cheese). Ironically, the people who would be the most motivated in ensuring that basic safety tools are used during every patient encounter are the least aware of their existence and importance.

MASTERING SAFETY HABITS

While no doctor questions the importance of precision in delivering, for example, radiation to a tumor, the idea that equal attention is necessary regarding handwashing can seem preposterous. This is the crux of the problem: eliminating instances of preventable harm depends on healthcare workers habitually using the very behaviors that can seem too simple to matter. Even among healthcare workers who are motivated to wash their hands consistently, achieving performance excellence can be difficult. Momentary lapses will occur. Equipping patients for their role in safe care has been the missing link in the industry's attempt to improve patient safety. When we finally prepare patients to speak up, we will sanction them as an important member of the healthcare team, and healthcare providers will have a far better chance of avoiding safety slips and lapses. This will require that providers convey the resounding message: "You are not challenging us. You are helping us."

In order to change the behavior of healthcare providers, we must influence the behavior of the patients around them. Thinking in terms of the Swiss Cheese Model, protective barriers can include things such as technology aids and training, but they can also involve the use of safety habits and routines. As showcased in recent best-selling books on habit change by Charles Duhigg and Gretchen Rubin, the science of behavior has proven that establishing and maintaining new habits is challenging, but doable. What healthcare has not appreciated is how essential patients are to the process.

Duhigg's book, *The Power of Habit*, draws on scientific research and countless examples from accomplished individuals and Fortune 500 companies to demonstrate how identifying a *keystone habit* can transform lives and organizations; the notion being that changing one critical behavior pattern often makes subsequent changes easier.

In the case of organizations, keystone habits are equivalent to essential routines. The process of forming habits or establishing organizational routines always necessitates that people identify triggers or *cues*, as well as rewards, that are associated with a desirable behavioral pattern; establish *routines* to perform in the presence of identified triggers or cues; and maintain a *belief* that change is possible. As Duhigg explains further, belief is the single most important aspect of the habit-formation process. That is, people must believe things will get better until they actually do get better. And they need a specific ritual, routine, or program to help them get there.[6]

In her book, *Better Than Before*, Rubin details why mastering desirable habits in our everyday lives (and work) is easier for some than for others. Nonetheless, she clarifies that *everyone* benefits when the environment provides signals (cues) that support people in doing exactly what they were already motivated to do. Without sufficient environmental stimuli, people will simply fail to achieve their desired behavioral patterns. This applies to changing behaviors that are highly individualistic (writing a few lines of poetry or practicing yoga every day) as well as those that have the potential to impact the broader society (reducing water consumption or increasing handwashing).[7]

Applying the analyses by Duhigg and Rubin to healthcare, there are two things that are not sufficiently abundant in hospitals today. First, *belief*: many healthcare workers have lost faith in their hospital's safety programs. In light of the field's dismal track record we can hardly blame them. Second, *cues and rewards*: too often the cues are missing that might serve as reminders to execute specific safety habits (or routines) at the critical moment of care. Why should we expect healthcare workers to always remember to use safety habits or routines that can seem too simple to matter when they are focused on a myriad of more complex care-delivery actions, get frequently interrupted, and are often tired from working long shifts? Likewise, there is rarely anyone present who has the wherewithal to acknowledge or express appreciation for (reward) providers when they do the right thing.

Consider that populating hospitals with well-informed patients who are capable of speaking up when lapses in safety protocols are observed would be tantamount to providing much-needed reminders or cues. And imagine how much easier it would be for healthcare workers to believe that success is possible knowing that the environment would be replete with friendly reminders to do the right thing with every patient every day during every encounter, and knowing that they would be reinforced for doing so.

NEW USE OF AN OLD TOOL

To a large extent, the idea of getting healthcare workers to do the right thing every day with every patient is asking them to cooperate with simple routines for the benefit of others. Two Harvard economists and two Yale psychologists recently conducted a review of field studies that examined factors that promote cooperation, noting this body of behavioral science research has a great deal to say about modifying habits for real-world solutions that require long-term behavior modification such as safety habits.[8] When it comes to getting people to cooperate to increase desired habits, the Ivy League researchers emphasized that financial incentives and material rewards often fail or even backfire, whereas leveraging social concerns that play on people's natural desire to be highly regarded by others are consistently effective.

This relates to what Garrett Hardin described as the *tragedy of the commons*, which refers to shared dilemmas wherein acts that benefit each individual cost the group as a whole. In his now classic paper, Hardin tells the story of herdsmen who were prone to overgraze cattle because each cattle brought them more money. However, each added cow also contributed to the destruction of the land, eventually destroying the land to the point that it was entirely unsuitable for grazing. In the end, everybody lost. The herdsmen never saw the tragedy coming because, for a long time, each received the full benefit of adding one more cow and suffered only a fraction of the cost of overgrazing. So each herdsman felt compelled to add one cow after another without taking stock of the fact that his actions, coupled with the actions of his fellow herdsmen, contributed to the depletion of the land.

Likewise, when it comes to pollution, the cost to the homeowner for purifying waste before dumping it into the river on his property might be greater than his share of the benefits for treating the discharged waste. Predictably, he will muddy the waters and worry about the downstream consequences when forced to later on, if this becomes necessary. It is a calculated risk, much like healthcare providers perceiving it is safe to skip handwashing a time or two or here and there without fully appreciating how their decisions contribute to the spreading of dangerous germs throughout the hospital.

As Hardin explains, when we are trying to get people to consistently do things that are in the best interests of the common good, more than they appear to be in our own best interests, it is foolish to expect a good outcome without somehow wiring the situation for compliance. Two things that help are observability and social norms. First, we can help establish compliance by making the desired action known to the people who would be most affected by the lack of it. In the case of healthcare-associated infections, then, patients must come to understand the risks they face when healthcare providers don't consistently wash their hands. But sometimes this is not enough.

In her 2015 book *Is Shame Necessary?* Jennifer Jacquet makes the case for why sometimes honor and shame must be invoked to motivate people to do the right thing. Although we tend to think of shaming as a deplorable act that is best left behind in the days when public hangings were in vogue, Jacquet shows how exposing people for deviating from established or desirable norms can be incredibly effective *but only if* it is used sparingly and in the right way. In proper form and measure, shame can be retrofitted as a powerful tool for bringing about the conformity that is essential to better long-term performance. When our own private guilt is not sufficiently strong to compel us to do the right thing, public exposure, or the mere fear of public exposure, can shame us into doing the right thing.

Retrofitted shame doesn't need to be too painful. In fact, when used properly, it focuses on the bad practice rather than a person's character. Done right, socially engineered shame simply and softly nudges people's behavior in the right direction by awakening a person's sense of moral obligation without inflicting undue humiliation. In the end, it helps us achieve our desired social norms. Moreover, in cases in which it is not possible to consistently punish transgressions in the usual ways, strategic use of retrofitted shame may be the only tool at our disposal.[9]

In the case of handwashing, it would be totally unfeasible to hire enough personnel to monitor providers' day-by-day and hour-by-hour bedside behavior to enforce compliance. The same is true for the safety behaviors that can avert or reduce off-the-mark procedures and medication administration errors. It would be much more pragmatic to prepare patients to recognize seemingly minor safety breaches and empower patients to nudge their providers to do the right thing. This also makes sense because the personal safety of patients is most at risk. Strategic use of soft shaming can be a particularly effective tool when dealing with behaviors that involve breaches that are so common people think of them as quasi-acceptable practices/quasi-errors—the "violations" that have been normalized because "everybody does it."

Logically, letting healthcare workers know how many of their peers signed a pledge to use specific safety habits, and to show appreciation when receiving reminders during momentary lapses, would represent a powerful use of "retrofitted shame" to establish more desirable safety norms. For shaming to work, it must hit the sweet spot, meaning it can be "too weak or too strong, too brief or too permanent."[10]

Sometimes all it takes to establish a more desirable norm is for people to know they are being watched. The *audience effect* might have a more powerful influence on human behavior than we give it credit, especially under circumstances in which the visual attention is coupled with a consequence for violating the social norm.[11] In fact, research has demonstrated that providers are more likely to comply with safety practices such as proper hand hygiene when they know their patients are watching them.[12] Furthermore, plenty of research has demonstrated the conditions under which patients are more likely to take action. Consistent with the *Health Belief Model*, patients are more likely to speak up for safety under conditions in which they perceive a threat to their health is serious, know what to do to help prevent being harmed, have confidence in their ability to do what is required, and believe the costs of speaking up are worth it.[13]

Bottom line: we cannot achieve the desired norms for patient safety unless the public becomes engaged in the process.

BOTCHED ATTEMPTS TO ENGAGE PATIENTS

Effective public or *community engagement* refers to the process of involving citizens in the decisions that affect their lives and mobilizing them for the purpose of undertaking activities to improve the conditions that affect them.[14] Within the healthcare arena, there has been growing appreciation for the idea of engaging patients to improve patient outcomes and satisfaction.[15] As noted by physician Donald Berwick, one of the pioneering and most renowned leaders of the patient safety movement, adopting a more patient-centered view of healthcare is essential; although, at first, it will necessitate some shifts in power and control from those who give care to those who receive it.[16] This process must begin by engaging with patients to understand how they view and value their role in the delivery of safe care.

Patient engagement refers to the idea that people must be invited to take action to obtain the greatest benefit from the healthcare services available to them.[17] To meet the Joint Commission's patient engagement goal, hospitals must "encourage the active involvement of patients and their families in the patient's own care as a safety strategy," and compliance is measured by whether or not hospitals define and communicate a way for patients and families to report concerns about safety and whether hospitals actually encourage them to do so.[18]

Initially, a lot of people in healthcare dismissed the idea of engaging and empowering patients to improve safety as a misguided and politically correct agenda.[19] They thought of it as a mere fluff-and-puff, touchy-feely strategy that had no real potential to improve outcomes. However, the evidence to support this idea exists and continues to grow.

For example, a large-scale survey of recently discharged hospital patients found that 91 percent believed they could help prevent medical errors; although patients varied with respect to their confidence or willingness to speak up about handwashing oversights, confirming their identity, and medication administration.[20] A patient education intervention in four hospitals in the United Kingdom led to about a 34 percent increase in soap usage by healthcare staff, regardless of the hospital's preintervention levels of soap usage.[21] Another UK handwashing intervention with hospitalized patients found that education improved their likelihood of speaking up—especially if the providers also wore a button that said, "It's OK to ask."[22] A 2008 review of the scientific literature found no journal article that addressed consumer involvement in patient safety initiatives in the United States or abroad. The review concluded that "evidence for consumer involvement in patient safety initiatives is limited and involvement of consumers is unlikely to occur without active recruitment programs."[23]

In the years since that review, many hospitals, healthcare systems, and government agencies have begun to more aggressively develop strategies to engage patients. To more effectively promote patient and family engagement in hospital settings, the Agency for Healthcare Research and Quality contracted the American Institutes for Research to review and report on the status of tools and practices that were currently in use. The review included team input, key informant interviews, and a comprehensive scan of the scientific and gray literature—including material available on 110 websites and 330 tools.[24]

In spite of the rapid expansion of literature and materials, the American Institutes for Research found they were universally inadequate to the task at hand. The institute identified four major gaps with existing patient-engagement efforts: the information was not attuned to patient and family member experiences; lacked concrete, actionable support for individual patients (and professionals) to engage in specific behaviors; omitted complementary strategies for patients and those who care for them; and failed to include specific guidance for hospitals to implement recommended engagement practices. Among the handful of tools with content deemed potentially useful, none was found to be ready for use in its current form. Low health literacy was identified as a significant barrier to the effectiveness of materials in print.[25]

Health literacy refers to a patient's ability to read, understand, and act upon health information. It requires more than the ability to read. It requires reading, listening, analytic, and decision-making skills, and the ability to apply such skills to health situations. Health literacy emphasizes the importance of clear communication between healthcare providers and their patients, recognizing that both the patient's and the provider's skills affect comprehension, and it is a dynamic construct that is affected by situational factors.[26] In addition to the choice of content (the amount of information or the complexity of information), health literacy can be compromised by design elements (small print, limited white space).[27]

Research has documented that regardless of their reading level, patients prefer medical information that is easy to read and understand.[28] For people who do not have strong reading skills, access to easy-to-read material is not just desirable, it is essential. Attending to content and design issues of patient advisories is critical because the average American reads at the ninth-grade level, while one in five American adults read at the fifth-grade level or below.[29] Yet most healthcare advisories have been written for above the tenth-grade level, leaving up to ninety million Americans unlikely to adequately comprehend existing materials.[30]

Over one-third of hospitalized Americans have low health literacy, which is not surprising because the problem is more acute among the elderly, minimally educated, and chronically ill populations[31]—the very people who are at increased risk for being hospitalized. In fact, more than two-thirds of Americans over the age of sixty and up to half of minority populations have literacy skills that may be either inadequate or marginal for comprehending existing patient-advisory pamphlets.[32] As such:

> Most of the literature on patient and family engagement roles focuses on what patients could do (or what researchers and policymakers want patients to do) instead of discussing what behaviors patients and family members currently engage or would be willing to engage during clinical encounters.[33]

Even among professionals who have been involved with the development of notable patient safety advisories, some openly doubt whether healthcare providers would regularly discuss the advisories with patients, reinforce the advisories' messages, or even support their use.[34]

Furthermore, the timing of the delivery of patient-oriented education has not been ideal. Because patients experience heightened states of anxiety during hospital stays, it is reasonable to expect the health literacy among all patients, including the highly educated, to plummet upon admission. Therefore, even with access to the best patient advisories, waiting until people are hospitalized as the primary way to encourage an active role in the delivery of safe care amounts to too little too late.[35] Introducing patients to safety expectations through written materials during or shortly before a hospitalization simply doesn't constitute genuine patient engagement.

Whereas greater patient (or consumer) engagement in US healthcare has been a matter of considerable discussion at a national level, hospitals have responded by branding and printing tons of materials directed at patients. But very few hospitals have actually engaged with the communities they serve to identify and implement realistic ways for patients to fully assert their rights and responsibilities as partners in safe care.

EMPOWERING PEOPLE TO SPEAK UP FOR SAFETY

Speaking up for safety refers to someone raising concerns for the benefit of safety and quality care upon becoming aware of risky or deficient action on the part of others.[36] Empowering people to speak up for safety is a challenge in every type of organization, and there is ample evidence to indicate that this represents a serious problem for the healthcare industry. Since 2007, hospitals around the country have been completing the Agency for Healthcare Research and Quality (AHRQ) Patient Safety Culture Survey. It allows hospitals to benchmark their culture against other hospitals. In 2011, over one thousand hospitals completed the survey, and AHRQ contracted an independent organization to examine the degree of improvement in the culture of safety among US hospitals from 2007 to 2011. The results indicated that there had been no overall progress, with half of the employees still saying they did not feel free to speak up for safety. They reported experiencing or fearing they would experience punitive responses from the administration for identifying and reporting errors, believing that reporting mistakes would be held against them and threaten their job security.[37]

If, after years of effort, healthcare employees still believe they cannot speak up for safety, why should we expect patients to do so? Actually, a 2014 review of the literature on studies that sought to increase people's ability to speak up for safety provides support for the idea. Authors of the comprehensive review determined that healthcare worker decisions to speak up are influenced by their degree of perceived *fear* of administrative retaliation (getting fired), *motivation* based on the extent to which they believe patient safety might be at risk, and *clarity* about the proper course of action (ambiguous versus clear-cut expectations).[38] Patients do not need to be worried about being fired by hospital administrators, which lays the first concern to rest. Public health–oriented campaigns could successfully address the other two issues (motivation and perceived risk). Such campaigns would also have the added advantage of focusing exclusively on simple, effective safety habits as opposed to more complex quality issues that require a myriad of judgment calls involving a high degree of uncertainty about correct actions. Of course, such campaigns must include complementary efforts to prepare providers to respond favorably when patients do speak up for safety.

Involving a community—patients, prospective patients, lay caregivers, patient advocates, and hospital visitors—to eliminate any one of healthcare's trifecta of current safety issues would constitute realistic and genuine patient engagement. The process would equip patients with a specific and important role as a member of their care team—the very thing that healthcare leaders have been seeking.

PUTTING IT ALL TOGETHER

Mastering safety habits is something every healthcare worker must do, something every patient wants them to do, and something the public can help them do. But how can this be achieved? In the process of gathering information for a comprehensive infection control and prevention project, Johns Hopkins conducted a brief pilot study to gain insights for improving handwashing compliance. Study results underscored the fact that getting patients to speak up for safety is not always easy. Staff collected information from patients in one of their outpatient clinics. Results of their face-to-face pilot survey revealed that 86 percent of patients indicated that they would be willing to be a hand-hygiene observer, although almost one-third fewer patients (56 percent) expressed a willingness to speak up if they saw a provider fail to use proper hand hygiene.[39]

Empowering patients to know when and how to take action is precisely the focus of many successful public health campaigns, but this is not what hospitals alone are prepared to do well. However, community-based coalitions, which typically include hospital-community partnerships, represent a well-established and proven method for engaging consumers in public health initiatives across a wide range of topics. Community-based coalition work arguably represents a missing component of a comprehensive framework for tackling the hospital safety crisis, especially for problems as prevalent, predictable, and preventable as those comprising the current hospital safety trifecta.

Whatever reasons have existed for treating hospital safety as an in-house matter, it is time to take this issue to the streets. Doing more of the same and expecting better results is not rational. Besides, the essential components of a successful public health campaign to improve patient safety have already been established, including:

- specific safety habits for eliminating or radically reducing common medical mistakes
- proven behavioral science principles to facilitate the mastery of safety habits
- experience using community coalitions to mobilize support for health-related behavioral changes across large groups of people and organizations.

Understanding the problem of patient safety within a broader public health framework that centers on patient engagement would represent a paradigm shift that supports the integration and application of knowledge from a number of fields—something that is evidently necessary. Recent testimonials on the Joint Commission's Center for

Transforming Healthcare's website speak to the value of a new paradigm of this nature.[40]

> The hand-hygiene initiative focuses attention on the problem of hand hygiene and offers an evidence-based way to measure the problem, implement interventions, and measure improvement. The challenge is making handwashing a habit that all healthcare workers do without even thinking about it.

—Linda Maragakis, MD, MPH, Johns Hopkins Medical Institutions

> We will know if we have been successful with the hand-hygiene initiative when we see the culture begin to change in our organizations. I hope that we will see people reminding each other to wash their hands, and those reminders will not be interpreted as punitive, but instead as teamwork.

—Beth Lanham, BSN, RN, Froedtert Hospital

> Transforming healthcare means taking what we have done; looking at it in a new way; taking it in a new direction; and, rather than making incremental improvement, making revolutionary improvement.

—Brian Regan, PhD, New York Presbyterian Healthcare System

The behaviors that are required to eliminate the most prevalent, predictable, and preventable hospital safety events represent what could become healthcare's keystone habits. Keystone habits are those that convey "success doesn't depend on getting every single thing right, but instead relies on identifying a few key priorities and fashioning them into powerful levers."[41] Once we figure out how to develop and sustain these habits, we will have gone a long way toward restoring confidence that it is possible to keep patients safe. Without them, we will continue to spin our wheels with too little progress for all the energy expended.

CHAPTER 3

Make It a Bad Day to Be a Bug
Prevent the Spread of Dangerous Infections

Johanna Daly

Johanna Daly was a healthy and active sixty-three-year-old woman when she slipped on an icy sidewalk when leaving a restaurant. She broke her shoulder and underwent a scheduled operation a few days later. The surgery and initial recovery went as planned. A young intern visited her hospital room to check the surgical incision. Without washing his hands or donning gloves, he removed her bandages and squeezed the incision. It looked good, and she was scheduled for discharge. Over the next few days, the surgical site became unbearably painful. Four days later, when seen in an emergency department, a physician drained over a quart of pus from the wound. It was necessary to schedule Johanna for emergency surgery to further clean the infected wound. It turned out that Johanna had contracted a virulent and antibiotic-resistant infection or "superbug" called MRSA (Methicillin-resistant Staphylococcus aureus, pronounced *mursa*). Being infected with MRSA led to a rapid decline in her health. Within days of the second surgery, Johanna's organs began to shut down and she was placed on a ventilator in an intensive care unit, where she remained until her death several months later.[1]

SUPERBUGS

Hundreds of people suffer similar fates as Johanna Daly every day. All of us are potential victims of healthcare-associated infections. These deadly bugs have long been known to lurk around inpatient facilities, especially hospitals, nursing homes, and rehabilitation centers. Of growing concern is that some of these infections involve *superbugs* that

are highly resistant to antibiotic treatment due to the widespread overuse of antibiotics. Sometimes these bugs are stronger than any weapon
we have to fight them.

Healthcare-associated infections may represent the most common
patient safety event, killing up to one hundred thousand US hospital
patients each year. And this is only the tip of the iceberg. This number
does not include the nearly two million people who are infected but
manage to survive—like NBA superstar Grant Hill. In 2003, this strong,
healthy, young athlete nearly died from a MRSA infection acquired in
the hospital during routine ankle surgery. The infection ate a hole in his
ankle, required a skin graft and an extended hospitalization, and was
followed by a six-month course of intravenous antibiotic treatment.

Furthermore, these superbugs are becoming common in outpatient
settings. A couple of years ago, I picked one up as a result of a brief
scoping procedure that was performed in an outpatient clinic. Being
in great health and not having been hospitalized, nobody expected me
to pick up a dangerous superbug that normally affects critically ill patients. In fact, the infection I contracted is a superbug that is commonly
referred to as an "ICU bug" because it is historically found only among
people being cared for in intensive care units.

I recovered, but it took a year of misguided treatment before the
unexpected source of my symptoms was discovered. Adding to my
frustration (and discomfort), appropriate treatment was delayed partly
because of the failure of a hospital laboratory to process a test and a
breakdown in communication between a hospital emergency department and a specialist—this occurred in spite of my attempt to prevent
such a mistake.

Unfortunately, this scenario is likely to play out frequently. Superbugs are now spreading beyond hospital walls and into outpatient care
settings. Scarier still, superbugs are creeping their way into community
settings, like locker rooms, classrooms, and daycare centers.

CLEAN CARE IS SAFE CARE

Many people think that eliminating healthcare-associated infections is
the sort of problem that requires expensive, high-tech solutions. We

certainly do have emerging tools like custom-engineered germ-killing counter surfaces and $100,000 robots that scan hospital rooms to kill detected germs.[2] The fact is, however, that the single most effective solution for preventing the spread of infection involves proper hand-washing—plain and simple.[3]

In short, *everyone*—providers, hospital support staff, visitors, and others—should wash their hands *every time* they enter and exit an ICU and every time they enter and exit any patient room. A successful national handwashing campaign would save many of the one hundred thousand lives that end every year due to healthcare-associated infections. It would also eliminate more than $150 million in avoidable healthcare expenditures.[4] Based on published data, an average two-hundred-bed hospital incurs over $1.7 million in annual MRSA infection expenses that are attributable to handwashing noncompliance. A mere 1 percent increase in hand-hygiene compliance can result in a savings of almost $40,000 per year for a two-hundred-bed hospital.[5]

SO, WHAT GIVES?

Proper hand hygiene could eliminate the vast majority of hospital-acquired infections (and associated human and financial costs), but after a decade of intense effort to establish consistent and proper hand hygiene, on average, only about 50 percent of doctors and nurses in leading hospitals wash their hands as needed.[6] Sometimes rates have been shown to be as high as 90 percent,[7] but experience proves that such findings tend to be inflated due to observation strategies that alert providers to when they are being monitored and reporting that is skewed by virtue of outcomes being tied to employee bonuses. At any rate, why is proper hand hygiene characteristically low? The problem is actually a complex one that healthcare has struggled with, to varying degrees, for hundreds of years.

A LITTLE HANDWASHING HISTORY

In *Get Me Out*, Randi Hutter Epstein recounts that in the early 1800s, many women died soon after childbirth from *childbed fever*, or what we now refer to as puerperal or postpartum infections. All sorts of theories circulated to explain why healthy women became gravely ill and all too often died after delivering their babies. It turned out that they were dying of what we now call healthcare-associated infections. The major source of their infections was the unclean hands of the doctors who cared for them.

At that time, many women who conceived children out of wedlock were prone to abandon or kill their newborns rather than suffer social retribution for bearing an out-of-wedlock baby. To curb this trend, free maternity clinics sprang up across Europe. Supervised medical and midwifery students staffed the clinics, enabling the free clinics to be used as training sites. There were two of these clinics in Vienna—one staffed largely by physicians and medical students, the other staffed by midwives and their trainees. If a woman delivered her baby in one of these clinics, the clinic would cover all medical expenses and arrange for the baby to be adopted.

Women wanted the free care for themselves and their babies but were afraid to deliver their babies in these clinics. So much so that they often preferred to deliver their babies in the dirty streets of Vienna because they were aware that the rate of childbed fever was lower among women who delivered babies in the streets rather than in the clinics. Some went so far as to feign spontaneous delivery right outside the clinic doors to reap the benefits of the free care without having to deliver their babies inside.

Interestingly, the death rate due to childbed fever was much higher in the physician-run clinics than the midwife-run clinics. Dr. Ignaz Semmelweis, a young resident physician, observed women begging to be admitted to the midwife clinic rather than the physician clinic. The women were frightened; Semmelweis was perplexed. What was the difference?

It eventually dawned on Semmelweis that most physicians performed autopsies while the midwives did not. Thus he concluded that the doctors were transferring particles from the cadavers to their obstetric patients.

Noting the dangers apparently associated with being cared for by the physicians, Semmelweis ordered medical students and doctors to wash their hands with a chlorinated lime solution when leaving the autopsy room and before caring for live patients. In very short order, he observed a 90 percent decrease in deaths associated with childbed fever. So, of course, across Europe a successful handwashing campaign took root and millions of lives were saved, right? Au contraire!

Semmelweis's conclusion that childbed fever was associated with a lack of cleanliness was highly controversial. Many physicians were appalled that he would suggest patient deaths were due to a lack of cleanliness on their part and refused to comply with his handwashing regimen. Although his theory was gaining traction in some communities, he was driven out of Vienna.

While practicing medicine in another city, Semmelweis continued his campaign to promote rigorous handwashing. He began to feel a frantic need to see such change implemented and wrote increasingly angry letters to prominent European obstetricians over the lack of compliance. At one point, he denounced some of his medical colleagues as "irresponsible murderers." Many of them, and eventually his wife, concluded he was losing his mind.

Semmelweis was then forcibly admitted to an insane asylum where he suffered from severe beatings by guards on duty. Some of his wounds became infected. In a distressing twist of fate, Semmelweis died fourteen days later of a institution-associated infection—just like the women he was trying to save from suffering the same misfortune.[8]

THE BEAT GOES ON

One hundred fifty years later, the battle rages on. A cadre of impassioned professionals continues to promote handwashing campaigns, resolved to put the knowledge into action with every patient, in every encounter, every time. Among the broader guild of physicians, there remains wide variability for the appreciation of the importance of proper hand hygiene.

Remember, safety training is typically mandatory for the employed hospital staff while remaining optional for physicians who work in the same facilities. As you would expect, physician participation in voluntary safety training is notoriously low. As a consequence, nurses and other staff often observe physician leaders failing to use safety practices that they themselves have been told are critically important. Over time, lack of physician buy-in corrodes employee commitment to behavior change. For many, the expected safety behaviors never become ingrained practices, and any initial gains in this direction are quickly lost.

Even when physician leaders are current on a hospital's patient safety guidelines, they sometimes inadvertently undermine a culture of safety through their own actions. When they don't do as expected, the ramifications are compounded. It is the physicians' behavior the staff tends to emulate—regardless of what policies are in place.

Case in point: during my first month as a patient safety director for a large healthcare system, I experienced the challenge of confronting someone about clean, safe care. According to policy, it was imperative that healthcare professionals wash their hands each and every time they enter and exit the intensive care unit. Making patient safety rounds with a hospital vice president (let's call her Dr. Drift) taught me an unintended lesson. Dr. Drift snapped when I reminded her to wash her hands upon exiting the intensive care unit. With irritation in her voice and in front of everyone present, she sniped, "I didn't touch any patients." Being brand-new to the field and my role, I hesitated, blushed, and wondered whether there was an exception to the rule of which I was unaware.

Fact: Dr. Drift had not touched any patients. However, she had worked on several computers in the unit, walked in and out of patient rooms, and greeted several people. Soon after this incident, I learned that MRSA bugs are capable of living on computer keyboards for up to six weeks. Of course, the physician needed to wash her hands!

In one fell swoop, Dr. Drift had undermined my authority and confidence as a new safety director. In effect, she sabotaged the hospital's patient safety program. Like Dr. Drift, hospital leaders unwittingly undermine the culture of safety in hospitals every day. This happens hundreds of times over among direct care providers. Such unsafe "exceptions" become "accepted" patterns, leading to a false sense of security and lack of personal ownership for the problem. Whatever initial safety gains are made after training, they can drift away ever so quickly.

I guarantee you that Dr. Drift thought of herself, and still thinks of herself, as a champion for patient safety in her hospital. Like so many other hospital administrators who set the tone for safety, she was experiencing the very sort of disconnect between an abstract concept and her personal actions. She knew the rule about washing hands before entering and after exiting the ICU, but she didn't think of herself as someone capable of spreading a lethal infection. Her mind quickly generated an exception to the rule, and she was annoyed for having her seemingly benign behavior challenged.

Interestingly, three years after this incident, my husband and I visited a friend in the intensive care unit at the very same hospital. I was shocked—but clearly shouldn't have been—that we were able to walk in and out of the hospital unit and in and out of our friend's room without any staff attending to whether we (or the multitude of my friend's visitors) washed hands. Signs were posted on the ICU door reminding people entering to wash their hands, but I, who no longer worked there, was the one who had to say something to protect our friend.

Believing that signage alone is sufficient to establish essential safety routines among hospital visitors is unrealistic. And the same can be said about expecting staff to have the ability or time to catch all visitors entering a unit and train them on proper handwashing.

THE GOOD NEWS

In spite of some persistent challenges, significant progress has occurred since Semmelweis's day and even over the last few years. There is virtual unanimity among today's healthcare professionals that proper hand hygiene is essential for preventing the spread of deadly healthcare-associated infections. We now have a set of established hand-hygiene standards for hospitals, and handwashing campaigns have been a focus of patient safety programs in most hospitals.

Yet the rate of healthcare-associated infections is still on the rise. In 2009, leaders of national patient safety organizations met to discuss this escalating problem. Their meeting signaled a new day when these leaders unanimously acknowledged the mounting evidence that virtually every healthcare-associated infection is preventable and that they could no longer be considered the "cost of doing business."[9]

Together, this prominent group of patient safety experts established the *Chasing Zero Consensus*, which refers to the idea that anything other than a goal of zero healthcare-acquired infections is unacceptable for hospitals today. Zero healthcare-associated infections was the agreed-upon goal because the knowledge exists to address this problem and the solutions are often quick, uncomplicated, and essentially cost-free.[10]

The zero-tolerance goal was not only revolutionary for healthcare; it was also necessary. As legendary football coach Vince Lombardi once said, "Perfection is not attainable. But if we chase perfection, we can catch excellence."

THE SWEET SMELL OF (A BIT OF) SUCCESS

Modern healthcare has proven that it has the capacity to radically reduce, if not effectively eliminate, this problem. Consider the case of the subset of healthcare-associated infections that are related to the insertion of central lines, called *central line infections*.

Central lines refer to long, thin, flexible tubes that are inserted through the skin of the arm or chest to make it easier to deliver medications and fluids over a long period of time or in large quantities. They are often used with patients requiring intensive care, cardiac treatment, dialysis, or chemotherapy. Use of central lines puts patients at increased risk for infections, including dangerous bloodstream infections that can lead to extended hospital stays or death.

These infections account for 15 percent of all healthcare-associated infections and 30 percent of infection-related deaths. They are also financially burdensome, costing up to $40,000 per case.[11] Recognizing the importance of eliminating these dangerous infections, Dr. Peter Pronovost from Johns Hopkins University led efforts to develop a straightforward checklist of steps for preventing central line infections. He and his colleagues ended up with a five-part checklist. Verifying that hands have been properly washed is one of the first tasks on the checklist.[12]

After establishing leadership support, Pronovost and his colleagues were able to establish 95 percent compliance with the checklist and eliminate nearly all central line infections in his hospital.[13] Healthcare leaders in Michigan decided to adopt the use of Pronovost's central line checklist statewide and secured federal funding to support the project. The results were amazing. Including all private and public hospitals in the state, Michigan was able to eliminate 70 percent of central line infections.[14] There is hope.

THE BAD NEWS

We still have a long way to go. The overall rate of healthcare-associated infections remains high, and the majority of US hospitals are not compliant with recognized industry hand-hygiene standards. Even in the best hospitals, physicians and nurses wash their hands less than half the time required, with compliance rates as low as 30 percent.

Again, why do the best doctors and nurses at some of the country's leading hospitals still only wash their hands half as often as prescribed? While handwashing sounds like a simple issue, it is actually a complex one. Most of us know when, how, and why we must wash our hands. The issue is not a lack of knowledge. The breakdown occurs in putting this knowledge into action with every patient, every time. There are obstacles in the way of full handwashing compliance at every level. As discussed earlier, too many hospitals still don't have a hand-hygiene policy in place, and policy represents only the first step in changing employee behavior.

TOO MUCH OF A GOOD THING?

The importance of handwashing is not at issue. What remains up for debate in the minds of providers is "How much is enough?" It is hard for most of us to believe that the amount of handwashing espoused by patient safety experts is really necessary. It can seem like overkill. To be compliant with policy guidelines, a provider would need to wash his hands many times a day and over a hundred times per week. In a hospital setting, where attention demands are high and the work pace is fast and the hours are long, by-the-book handwashing could come to feel like too much of a good thing. But new research shows that increasing compliance from mediocre to high rates is not enough. Gains are still realized by getting compliance above 95 percent.[15]

The sheer number of handwashing episodes required in a day represents an obstacle in and of itself. Anything that we need to remember twenty to sixty—or even one hundred—times a day is likely to be missed a time or two. Nobody is perfect. The spell-check factor, as described by Megan McArdle in her book, *The Up Side of Down*—can spell disaster for patients.

> We all go through our lives making a constant string of mistakes, but because nothing bad happens, we're barely even aware of them. . . . The most dangerous thing about the Spell-Check Factor is that we forget it's there; we don't register all the times that we have come close to making fatal mistakes. That one moment when a doctor decides not to wash her hands almost never kills anyone. But millions of such moments kill tens of thousands of people every day.[16]

In fact, more than one in every twenty-five US hospital patients is dealing with a healthcare-associated infection on any given day, but very few of these are ever traced back to the providers who spread them.[17] Intellectually, healthcare workers know hand hygiene prevents infections and saves lives. However, when a worker touches a MRSA-ridden surface and spreads the microscopic bugs around the hospital, he never knows it. "When your mistakes rarely lead to a bad outcome, you lose the necessary feedback that helps you improve."[18] However, as explained by the Swiss Cheese Model and showcased in chapter 7, serious safety events are almost always preceded by a stream of minor errors.

The situation is compounded by the fact that, until recently, healthcare-associated infections were accepted as an unavoidable cost of doing business. Countless providers continue to hold this fatalistic belief. When healthcare-associated infections do befall their patients, many healthcare workers chalk it up to a fate to be expected of people with compromised immune systems. They certainly don't connect any instance of hand-hygiene noncompliance with their patients' illnesses.

Without clear feedback connecting actual behaviors with negative consequences, behavior change is not intuitive. Without the ability to connect their handwashing lapses with the lives they affect, providers go on infecting more and more people. The solution requires a shift from the focus on provider behavior and patient outcome to a focus on the process of getting things right. In other words, the process of washing hands must be an outcome in and of itself because providers cannot connect their individual actions with the rate of infection in their hospitals.

TAKING IT TO THE STREET

When providers and patients finally appreciate the full ramifications that not washing hands has for all of us, we will find a way to make consistent handwashing the norm rather than the exception. Because healthcare-associated infections are now spreading beyond the hospital walls, we must engage our patients. When it comes to hand hygiene in healthcare, we all need frequent reminders to do the right thing. For this to occur, patients en masse must be invited to be part of the solution. A successful public health campaign will not only raise awareness among patients about the importance of proper hand hygiene but will also provide actions that everyone can take to ensure safer care for themselves and their loved ones.

BUILDING BLOCKS FOR A PUBLIC HEALTH HANDWASHING CAMPAIGN

If the public is going to be inundated with information about proper hand hygiene in healthcare settings, providers need to be ready for this change. They must be prepared to appreciate reminders from patients to wash hands and to graciously respond to patient requests. To facilitate this process, we need to develop public education that includes tools and language that most any provider, patient, and lay caregiver can and will use. When it comes to behaviors like handwashing—the potentially life-saving behaviors that seem too simple to matter—we need powerful reminder tools that are meaningful to everyone on the team. Effective reminders are what we call *sticky messages*—brief phrases or jingles that once learned are easily remembered. Sticky messages are short but convey a lot.

The tables below contain information to promote consistent handwashing. Table 3.1 summarizes key points from this chapter; table 3.2 is a checklist patients can use to ensure they are adequately and timely prepared to advocate for their safety; and table 3.3 provides sample language that patients and providers can reference as they think about speaking up for safety and reinforcing others when they do so. Table 3.3 includes a "sticky message" to help people remember when they are supposed to wash their hands. (See *Made to Stick* by Chip and Dan Heath[19] to learn more about crafting messages that people are likely to remember.)

Tables 3.1 and 3.3 are offered merely as examples of the sort of information that can be adapted for use in educational campaigns, public service announcements, hospital and clinic brochures, encounter summaries generated by electronic health records, and other relevant community venues. As described in chapter 6, such material should be tailored to its target audience.

Table 3.1.

WHAT YOU NEED TO KNOW Healthcare-Associated Infections
Information for Patients
Every year, one hundred thousand hospital patients die as a result of infections that they pick up in US hospitals. Healthcare-associated infections are dangerous, but preventable. Proper handwashing is the single most effective way to stop the spread of these infections. Doctors and nurses wash their hands less than half the times required. In the hustle and bustle of delivering care, it is easy to have a momentary lapse. Even the best providers need reminders to wash their hands. It is important that all providers (and visitors) wash their hands every time they enter or exit a patient room—everyone must wash on the way in, and wash on the way out. We are all part of the healthcare team. Don't be afraid to remind your healthcare providers and visitors to wash their hands when you don't see it happen with your own eyes. Speaking up for safety is not about challenging our providers, it is about helping them. By working together, we can prevent people from picking up harmful and potentially deadly hospital infections. In the hospital and other healthcare settings, it's okay to ask everyone to wash their hands on the way in and out of patient rooms. Everyone must "wash in" and "wash out," and most people need help remembering to do so.
Information for Providers
More than one out of every twenty-five US hospital patients is dealing with a healthcare-associated infection on any given day. Proper handwashing is the single most effective way to stop the spread of these infections. Without realizing it, we all go through our lives making a constant string of mistakes; however, we barely notice most of them because the *spell-check factor* kicks in: We don't register all the times we make what could become a significant mistake. For example, the moment we decide not to wash our hands never immediately kills anybody, but millions of such moments kill patients every day. Because such minor mistakes rarely lead to a bad outcome, we lose the necessary feedback to motivate us to improve. To overcome the spell-check factor, we need frequent reminders to wash hands every time we enter and exit a patient room. Patients can help us remember to "wash in" and "wash out." However, we must actively encourage patients to do so and respond approvingly when they do.

Table 3.2.

PATIENT ACTION PLAN Healthcare-Associated Infections		
TIMING	**PATIENT ACTION**	**✓**
Before going to the hospital	I realize that I can help reduce the chance of getting a dangerous infection from the hospital.	
	I know why healthcare providers should wash their hands every time they enter and exit my room or examine me.	
	I understand how easy it is for hospital staff to forget to wash their hands.	
	I am ready to observe whether people wash their hands when they enter and leave my hospital room.	
	I practiced what to say if doctors, nurses, or anybody else forgets to wash their hands.	
	I explained to family and friends who will be involved in my care that speaking up is not about challenging healthcare professionals, it's about helping to keep all of us safe.	
	I know I can keep a bottle of hand sanitizer in my hospital room to remind myself and others about proper handwashing.	
While I am in the hospital and able to do so	I will remind my visitors to wash their hands when they enter and leave my room—to "wash in" and "wash out."	
	I will ask healthcare providers to wash their hands when I don't see it happen with my own eyes.	
	I might keep a bottle of hand sanitizer on my tray table as a helpful reminder.	

Table 3.3.

WHAT YOU CAN SAY	
When Someone Walks into a Patient Room without Washing Hands	
Sticky Message: Wash In, Wash Out	
Patient Request	**Desired Response**
"Sorry, I didn't see you wash your hands. I know it's important and I'd really appreciate you doing this for everyone's benefit."	*Staff*: "I just washed my hands before coming in, but I am happy to do it again for you to see. Thank you for speaking up."
"Hi, I'm so glad you're here. To make sure I don't pick up an infection, everybody needs to clean their hands before they come in my room. Do you mind washing yours?"	*Visitor*: "Oh, sure, no problem."
"Gee, I didn't see you wash your hands. I know you're busy, but I don't want anybody to pick up an infection. I'd feel better if I saw you wash your hands."	*Staff or Visitor*: Of course. Thank you for reminding me. It's people like you who keep us all safe."

CHAPTER 4

Oops!
Eliminate Mistakes during Surgery and Other Procedures

Removal of the Wrong Testicle

Benjamin Houghton had undergone successful treatment for testicular cancer. However, the treatment led to painful tissue damage. Being in his forties and the father of four, Mr. Houghton was scheduled for surgery to remove the painful testicle and elected to have a vasectomy on the other testicle. The hospital rescheduled the surgery several times. The day the surgery was finally performed, the usual consent form was presented. However, Mr. Houghton was reluctant to sign the form because he could not read the consent without his glasses. The staff assured him that it was the same form he had signed previously. In reality, the updated form had been completed improperly. The new consent form indicated that the right testicle was to be removed instead of the left. In accordance with the unverified (and incorrect) consent form, the wrong testicle was removed. As a result of his only healthy testicle being removed, Mr. Houghton was left with a choice between lifelong drug treatment that included serious risk for cancer and heart disease or a life without the drugs that would leave him with an inability for normal sexual functioning and risks for osteoporosis, broken bones, fatigue, memory loss, weight gain, loss of muscles strength, and depression.[1]

THE NATURE (AND NAME) OF THE BEAST

Mr. Houghton's experience of having the wrong testicle removed is a classic example of what medical literature describes as a *wrong-site surgery* and what this book refers to as an *off-the-mark procedure*. The two terms refer to exactly the same type of events, but the Joint Commission's term is confusing because it leads people to think that this category of events only pertains to surgeries. That is simply not the case.

The original term also led many to think of wrong-*site* surgeries as wrong-*side* surgeries. This sound-alike/look-alike problem has contributed to healthcare professionals overlooking events that involved the correct side of the body but the wrong location (e.g., correct arm but wrong location on the arm; correct hand, but wrong finger; etc.). The term has also caused some to overlook events involving the wrong patient or procedure. Although there has been a great deal of misunderstanding stemming from the original label choice, its definitional criteria are quite clear. As indicated in the table below, a wrong-site surgery/off-the-mark procedure includes any invasive procedure, including, but not limited to, surgery, which involves one of the four Ps: wrong patient, procedure, part, or place.

Furthermore, off-the-mark procedure criteria apply regardless of where the event occurs, who performs the procedure, and the degree of harm to a patient, including the absence of harm. For example, if

Table 4.1.

What Counts as an Off-the-Mark Procedure	
Type of Services	▪ Skin penetration through incision or needle ▪ Fluid or substance injected into a joint or body space ▪ Aspiration of body fluid or removal of body tissue ▪ Insertion of an instrument into a body opening or cavity ▪ Surgery
Type of Error	▪ Wrong *patient* ▪ Wrong *procedure*—other than indicated or intended (even if the procedure helped) ▪ Wrong body *part* (site)—symmetrical body parts such as legs, arms, feet ▪ Wrong body *place* or spot (site)—such as a bone's front vs. back, middle vs. end
No Exceptions	
❖ Any degree of harm, including the absence of notable harm to the patient ❖ Any type of facility—hospital, nursing home, outpatient surgery center, etc. ❖ Any type of provider—physician, nurse, technician, etc.	
An off-the-mark procedure refers to the same category of event as a wrong-site surgery, and it includes the exact same criteria set forth by the Joint Commission. The term *off-the-mark procedure* is offered as a substitute because the original term has contributed to widespread confusion about what constitutes an event.	

a lab technician drew blood from the wrong patient and this did not result in harm to anybody, the incident would still count as a wrong-site surgery/off-the-mark procedure. There are numerous reasons for tracking all such events regardless of the degree of harm, as will be explained later in this chapter.

THINGS THAT SHOULD NEVER HAPPEN

In the minds of most people, wrong patient, wrong part, wrong place, and wrong procedure mix-ups should *never* happen.[2] Indeed, the National Quality Forum includes this category of event among its list of what it literally calls *never events*, referring to, as the name implies, a healthcare behavior or patient outcome that should never occur.[3] The reason that off-the-mark procedures should never happen is they carry a high probability of a devastating outcome and are largely, if not completely, preventable. Well-publicized cases make clear why off-the-mark procedures are thought of as disturbing events that should never happen. They potentially signal that larger systemic problems exist. Consider these illustrative cases.

Wrong Leg Amputation: The Willie King Case

The widely publicized case of Willie King unleashed a flood of previously unreported off-the-mark procedures and drew modern medicine's attention to this category of events. The fifty-two-year-old Mr. King was admitted to University Community Hospital in Tampa, Florida, to have his leg amputated. During the procedure, the wrong leg was removed. By the time the surgeons realized their mistake, it was too late to reverse the damage caused, and the leg had to be removed. The attending surgeon was fined $10,000, and his medical license was revoked for six months. The hospital paid Mr. King $900,000, and the surgeon personally paid him another $250,000. The hospital admitted that a chain of errors culminated in the wrong leg being prepped for the surgery.[4]

Wrong Embryo Implant: The Susan Buchweiz Case

In a more recent case with a more complex outcome, a Californian by the name of Susan Buchweiz was awarded $1 million in damages to

settle a malpractice lawsuit against a fertility specialist who accidentally implanted her with the wrong embryos and hid the mistake until
her baby was ten months old. But the tragedy did not end there. The
embryos Susan Buchweiz received were intended for a married couple
that underwent in-vitro fertilization on the same day using the husband's
sperm and a different egg donor. The sperm donor was subsequently
granted temporary visitation rights, forcing coparenting among unfamiliar people. Later, the sperm donor and his wife sued for custody of the
three-year-old child that Buchweiz had raised since birth.[5]

Wrong Sperm Insemination: The Baby Jessica Case

A fertility clinic in New York impregnated Nancy Andrews with the
sperm of a complete stranger rather than the sperm of her husband. Instead of giving birth to a child that resembled both of her Caucasian parents, she delivered Baby Jessica who was significantly darker skinned.
Subsequent DNA testing revealed that Baby Jessica's biological father
was of African American descent. Although the Andrews have kept
Jessica and are raising her as their own, the couple has filed a medical
malpractice suit against the fertility clinic and against the embryologist
who reportedly mistakenly switched the samples.[6]

Wrong Organ Transplants: The Jésica Santillán Case

Seventeen-year-old Jésica Santillán awaited and was finally scheduled
to receive the heart and lungs of a patient whose blood type matched
hers. When the organs arrived, Jésica's physicians and surgical team
failed to check that the blood types actually matched. They did not.
As soon as the incompatible match between blood types was noticed,
the hospital acknowledged the error to Jésica's family, admitted that
simple errors contributed to the mistake, and committed to learning
from this horrible incident. Through concerted effort and extraordinary
means, the hospital was able to quickly obtain a second set of organs
for Jésica. But it was too late. Complications arose as surgeons attempted to replace the initial transplanted organs with the second set of
organs. Jésica was left in a comalike state and pronounced brain dead
soon thereafter. The hospital reached an agreement on an undisclosed
settlement with the family, which prohibits the hospital and family
from commenting further on the case.[7]

Admittedly, the experiences in Mr. Houghton's and these other cases probably represent some of the most horrifying examples of off-the-mark procedures; not all events in this category end with such a devastating impact. However, more than perhaps any other type of medical mistake, off-the-mark procedures are likely to harm both the patient and his or her providers. Even in the cases of minimal or no physical harm to patients, they often precipitate a loss of trust on the part of the patient and a loss of confidence on the part of the providers.

MINOR MIX-UPS BEGET MAJOR SCREW-UPS

If you wonder how a major or invasive procedure can go so terribly wrong, imagine this: a surgeon approaches the start of his day with the mindset that he has three big procedures that he has specifically planned and prepared for and a few mundane surgeries to perform. He goes through the usual routine of confirming with patients the procedures to be performed, including verification of the proper site of their operations. But then—as so often happens—there are a few snafus. Among other things, due to an overflow of cases and scheduling pressures, the patient on whom he will ultimately perform the wrong surgery—his last patient of the day—gets reassigned to a different operating room with a different surgical team. This means that the nurse who had performed the preoperative brief with the surgeon is no longer on the case. Instead, a new team is assembled to assist the surgeon. The surgery is completed successfully. However, fifteen minutes later, while dictating the operation report, the surgeon realizes he performed the wrong procedure on his last patient.

This case really happened. The surgeon immediately apologized to the patient. Although the surgeon convinced the patient to allow him to take her back into surgery to perform the correct procedure, she would not see him for follow-up care. According to her son, she had lost confidence in the surgeon. Having been emotionally traumatized by the experience, the surgeon, David Ring of Massachusetts General Hospital, felt compelled to shed more light on the problem of off-the-mark procedures. In 2010, he published an account of his unfortunate case in the *New England Journal of Medicine*.[8] Dr. Ring's write-up represents one of the rare instances in which a physician elected to publicly disclose his error before any press scrutiny or impending media attention.

As noted by surgeon John Clarke of Drexel University, off-the-mark procedures don't "just happen." However, minor mix-ups happen all the time, and it is precisely these errors that set the stage for major screw-ups. Scheduling errors are notorious for contributing to major downstream mistakes. Case in point: during the course of writing this chapter, a medical office assistant attempted to schedule me for a left knee MRI rather than a right knee MRI, which might have been understandable given that I was having issues on both sides of my body. I caught and corrected the error—or so I thought. Apparently, the office assistant's notes were confusing. When someone subsequently called from the MRI office to confirm my appointment, she had listed me for an MRI of both knees. Even if both knees had been subjected to this unnecessary diagnostic procedure, it would not have been such a terrible thing. And I could have easily assumed that the surgeon changed his mind and decided after my office visit to order an MRI of both knees— either for comparison purposes or because I had also been experiencing minor difficulty with my left knee. But this is the very sort of mix-up that could easily have contributed to a surgery on a healthy knee. That would have been a big deal! Interestingly, when I went to my first postsurgical physical therapy appointment, the clinician assigned to my case was also confused about which knee had been operated on, at first treating the wrong leg. Clearly, the initial error had lived on.

Here is another example of how easily an off-the-mark procedure might occur. Imagine that a nurse marks a left leg with an "L" to indicate the location for the preoperative injection of dye while another nurse marks the same leg with an "L" in a different spot to indicate where the surgery is to occur. If the surgeon only sees one marking, he or she could easily operate on the wrong area of the leg. Or, thinking back to Mr. Houghton's case, somebody could easily take the consent verification process for granted and mistakenly direct the surgeon to operate on the wrong side of the body. Such mix-ups happen too frequently.

The bottom line is there are innumerable ways for minor errors to contribute to harmful off-the-mark procedures. This is precisely why the Joint Commission focuses on all off-the-mark procedures regardless of how minor they are in terms of their impact on patients. Healthcare leaders need to learn about as many as possible so they can search for patterns that warrant widespread attention.

TOO COMMON FOR COMFORT

You may think of surgery being performed on the wrong patient to be one of the most unlikely types of medical error. Indeed, the occurrence of these events is rare compared to the frequency of healthcare-associated infections and medication administration errors,[9] but wrong-patient surgeries account for a substantial portion of off-the-mark procedures. A study based on hospital-based off-the-mark procedures for the state of Colorado identified twenty-five instances of wrong-patient operations over a six-year period.[10]

Initially, these numbers might sound pretty good. However, they are more concerning than you may realize. For one thing, the lead author of the Colorado study considered the numbers to be low and misleading. Concurring with this assessment, a professor of surgery and public health at Johns Hopkins University said that catastrophic surgical errors are "a lot more common than the public thinks," noting further:

> Each hospital, whether they publicly admit it or not, and whether or not it's discoverable in a lawsuit, has an episode of wrong-site or wrong-patient surgery either every year or once every few years. Almost every surgeon has seen one.[11]

Other research has documented anywhere between 1,300 and 4,000 off-the-mark procedures per year in US hospitals.[12]

The American healthcare system began systematically studying the problem of off-the-mark surgeries in the mid to late 1990s when the Canadian Orthopedic Association and then American Academy of Orthopedic Surgeons endorsed educational campaigns to prevent such mishaps. Around the same time, in 1997, the American Academy of Orthopedic Surgeons launched a voluntary "Sign Your Site" campaign, which encouraged surgeons to initial or otherwise mark the patient's body on the spot where the surgery was to occur. Nonetheless, this has not been a robust or popular area of patient safety research.

The relatively few studies that have been conducted only focused on operating room surgeries, and many of these studies have been further restricted to include only wrong-side surgeries (rather than the broader group of wrong person, procedure, part/place procedures and surgeries). These limitations create artificially low prevalence estimates of hospital-based off-the-mark procedures and say nothing about the presumably more common problem of off-the-mark procedures that occur in freestanding surgical centers where, with increasing frequency, invasive procedures are performed.

Regardless of the true prevalence of off-the-mark procedures, their occurrence in hospital and surgical centers is far too common for comfort. This is especially true considering that by 2004 surgeons were performing 230 million major surgeries per year. That figure amounts to one major surgery for every twenty-five human beings on the planet,[13] with American surgeons performing more than fifty million operations annually and American patients undergoing an average of seven operations in their lifetime.[14]

WHERE THERE'S SMOKE, THERE'S FIRE

The most minor off-the-mark procedures can, and usually do, signal a more serious problem. In this sense, they are sentinel events that signal things are not right. They warn us to look out for signs of danger just as would a guard on a sentinel tower. They signal "where there's smoke, there's fire."

When the Joint Commission notices a pattern of reported events, it issues a Sentinel Event Alert. These alerts describe high-risk conditions and underlying causes that are common across the reported events. To date, the Joint Commission has issued fifty-four Sentinel Event Alerts to help healthcare organizations determine their need to design new or redesign existing processes to avoid never events or similar problems, including off-the-mark procedures (wrong-site surgeries) as a sentinel event.

Without appreciation for the need to actively find and fix root causes of error (as opposed to incidentally discovering and fixing mistakes), it is easy to end up playing a game of whack-a-mole—a piecemeal or superficial attempt to solve a problem, resulting in only temporary or minor improvement. For example, this could amount to reprimanding or reassigning a surgical team member whose error contributed to an outcome involving patient harm, only to do so again with the new team member. Or, a whack-a-mole approach could entail repeatedly catching and addressing a scheduling error at the last minute in the preoperative area rather than finding a way to ensure that all the requisite information gets to the operating room scheduler in time to confirm all essential information. Falling short of finding and fixing the cause of the delayed paperwork leaves critical details to be attended to on the day of surgery and increases the likelihood of an off-the-mark procedure.

You might think that a hospital would get to the root of the problem after a high-stakes failure like any of the off-the-mark cases discussed so far, but that is not necessarily the case. It is just so much easier to "see" what went wrong at the pointy end of care and then to overlook the blunt end issues that led to the error in the first place. Rather than viewing a failure as the smoke that signals a burning fire somewhere else, people have a tendency to conclude that mistakes represent isolated incidents that can be addressed through individual and/or idiosyncratic measures. But the Swiss Cheese Model discussed in chapter 2 makes clear that this is rarely the case. System failures—also known as blunt end factors—almost always precede human error at the pointy end of care.

ONE HOSPITAL, ONE YEAR, THREE OFF-THE-MARK BRAIN SURGERIES

In 2007, a hospital was reported to have performed three brain surgeries on the wrong side of patients' heads—all within the span of a year. One patient died; the others survived despite having had their skulls cut and brains unnecessarily exposed in an extra place. In one case, a nurse observed the mistake but didn't speak up. In another, the nurse alerted the surgeon to lack of documentation about which side needed the operation, but the surgeon told her that he remembered which side was involved. The nurse questioned him again, but he insisted that he remembered correctly. So, she let it go. After these two cases, the hospital was ordered to make changes to prevent recurrences. But soon thereafter, a third case occurred. This prompted the state health department to dig deeper and discover that although the hospital had made some improvements within the operating room environment, these changes were insufficient. They had not spread to the rest of the hospital, leaving room for errors outside the operating room to contribute to the problem. The state's Department of Health reprimanded the hospital and fined it $50,000, and the story hit the press.[15]

Not long before these three off-the-mark procedures, surgeons at the same hospital operated on the wrong part of a child's mouth during a cleft palate surgery. And five months before that, one of the hospital's surgeons operated on the wrong finger of a patient. Although this story might have you thinking this happened in a third-rate hospital in rural America—you'd be wrong. These events happened at Rhode Island Hospital, a teaching hospital affiliated with the medical school at Brown University—an Ivy League institution—that is staffed by the best and brightest physicians. If it could happen there, it can happen anywhere.

According to the Joint Commission, there was a sense among the surgeons at the hospital that "I'm very well trained. I've done this procedure one hundred times. It's not going to happen to me." In addition to the arrogance and overconfidence of the physicians, the hospital's operating room nurses had become too timid to speak up and hold their ground when they saw safety issues. The end result was that the hospital had become a place where carelessness about small—though critical—details prevailed.[16]

After its run on serious off-the-mark procedures, Rhode Island Hospital took more comprehensive action to minimize the chance of more errors. But what if the hospital had viewed its first off-the-mark surgery as an important "smoke signal" and diligently searched to find and fix the cause of the error? In all likelihood, none of the wrong brain surgeries would have occurred. This problem plays out more often than we care to think.

Although communication breakdowns and scheduling glitches are common causes of off-the-mark procedures, the operating room milieu is a contributing factor in almost every case. It also has been well documented that nurses in hospitals across the country and abroad routinely experience physician arrogance, intimidation, and bullying. Consider this conversation that occurred in an operating room in October 2012.[17]

> *Surgeon* [Standing to the right of a patient under general anesthesia for hernia repair]:
>
> "Which side is the hernia?"
>
> *Assisting surgeon*: "I don't know. I did not see the patient."
>
> *Surgeon*: "Who saw the patient?"
>
> *Assisting surgeon*: "The house surgeon from the previous shift."
>
> *Surgeon*: "What does it say in the notes and consent?"
>
> *Assisting surgeon*: "Hernia repair, obviously."
>
> *Surgeon* [in anger]: "Obviously! But which bloody side?"
>
> There were a large group of people in that operation room: junior nurses and medical students and other staff. None of them will speak to the chief surgeon unless they are spoken to. Silence continued for a few moments.
>
> *Surgeon* [in exasperation]: "Does anybody know the side?"
>
> Medical student puts her hand up.
>
> *Surgeon* [very impatiently]: "Tell us. What are you waiting for?"
>
> *Medical student*: "I don't know for sure, but I was standing on the right of the patient's bed when I examined him and I had to reach out across to feel the hernia. So it must be on the left side."
>
> *Surgeon*: "Left it is then. Let us get this done."

The surgical team was lucky that day. The medical students had seen two other hernia preop patients the same day and fortunately they all had left groin hernias.[18]

We know that simply telling nurses and other personnel to speak up for safety doesn't work, but getting staff to speak up for safety is critically important to prevent safety mishaps. So, what can be done to prevent the continued accumulation of tragic off-the-mark stories?

Actually, there already exists a straightforward strategy for expediting the sort of communication among surgical teams that is essential for creating a situation in which it is safe to speak up for safety. Remember, people often talk about attitude affecting performance, which is, indeed, true; however, as psychological research has shown, it is sometimes easier to act oneself into a new way of thinking than to think oneself into a new way of acting. Providing a specific behavioral script can help hardwire desirable habits, often serving as the turnkey to behavior change. Healthcare already has an effective tool in its arsenal that accomplishes this. It's a checklist called the *Universal Protocol*.

THE UNIVERSAL PROTOCOL

The Universal Protocol represents the culmination of work by the World Health Organization (WHO) to improve surgical safety. In 2002, in the face of worldwide evidence of substantial public health harm due to inadequate patient safety, the WHO assembly adopted a resolution urging countries to strengthen their monitoring of patient safety events. Two years later, it launched the World Health Alliance for Patient Safety, which brought together heads of agencies, policymakers, and patient advocacy groups from around the world. The purpose of this alliance is to concentrate actions around focused patient safety topics. In 2005, the alliance chose healthcare-associated infections as its Global Patient Safety Challenge, and in 2007 it chose surgical safety as its second Global Patient Safety Challenge.

The World Health Alliance for Patient Safety selected Dr. Atul Gawande, a Harvard surgeon and popular writer, to lead the charge to improve surgical safety—an undertaking that involved experts from around the world who reviewed data and input from over fifty countries and over 280 million surgeries.[19] In his book *The Checklist Manifesto*, Gawande details the public health and political process of creating the Universal Protocol.

Through thoughtful testing and revising, the Universal Protocol became a meticulously crafted checklist. National and international groups have vetted the Universal Protocol for use in every operating room and venue where invasive procedures occur. This tool is a specific behavioral script that is believed to be capable of eliminating the majority (if not all) of off-the-mark procedures.[20] The beauty of this checklist is that it has balanced brevity and effectiveness, taking as few as two minutes to complete and, yet, capturing the critical elements for eliminating off-the-mark procedures.

The checklist is segmented into three distinct time-out processes— a preprocedure verification time-out, a site-marking time-out, and a preincision time-out. The first two time-outs occur with the active involvement of the patient (if possible) or the patient's lay caregiver or advocate. First, the preprocedure verification time-out is performed. It creates the need to confirm the correct patient, procedure, and site (body part and place). This occurs before the patient receives any anesthesia—except under emergency surgery conditions when this is not feasible or when even minor delays could mean the difference between life and death.

Second, the site verification time-out occurs. The licensed practitioner who is ultimately accountable for the procedure to be performed must mark the site of the surgery or procedure, obtaining confirmation from the patient. This process underscores the need for patients to be explicitly informed about the plan of their care. If, for example, a patient is eventually going to have both knees operated on but at different points in time, it can be critically important to understand which one is going to be addressed first. The surgeon could operate on the right knee but insert a left knee replacement part. You might think this is absurd, but it happens with too much regularity. When the patient's body is marked to indicate the site of the procedure, the marking must be unambiguous and made with ink that is visible and durable throughout the procedure.[21]

Then, after all preprocedure and site verification questions have been resolved, a third time-out is performed. This occurs prior to making the first cut. Other than the patient, who is often anesthetized by this point, the time-out must actively involve all members of the procedure team, including the person or persons performing the procedure, individuals providing anesthesia, the circulating nurse, and operating room technicians. In any hospital of reasonable size, it is fairly common for teams of clinicians who do not know each other to work together. For example, in the hospital where Gawande operates, there are forty-two operating rooms staffed by over one thousand nurses, technicians, residents, and physicians who rotate constantly. So team familiarity and collegiality cannot be taken for granted. Rather, a sense of team must be purposefully generated, even if it lasts only for the duration of a given procedure.

We know from psychological research that people who do not know each other's names generally do not work together nearly as well as those who do. Research has verified that the Universal Protocol's process of having people introduce themselves by name and role prior to the initiation of a procedure dramatically increases the sense of teamwork among surgeons, anesthesiologists, and nurses.[22] Anecdotal reports also confirm that this "team huddle" improves the likelihood that team members feel free to speak up for safety in the operating room environment. This seemingly simple behavioral routine of having team members introduce themselves before the procedure begins helps to overcome the silent disengagement that pervades many operating environments. This process minimizes the dangerous silo mentality of "that's not my problem."[23]

Finally, all team members must agree they have identified the correct patient, correct procedure, and correct site. This preincision process explicitly invites—actually requires—everyone on the team to speak before the procedure begins.

A DOUBLE-EDGED KNIFE AND ITS DOUBLE STANDARD

Surgery is a high-stakes endeavor, and surgeons endure years of training and grueling schedules before they are granted the authority to brutally invade the human body, bringing it to the brink of death in the hopes of healing and curing their patients. The chutzpah and drive that surgeons possess (or develop) to sustain them through such arduous training emboldens them to initiate and oversee life-threatening procedures on a daily basis. At the same time, their brass necks can undermine their willingness to admit they are fallible and to own their mistakes. Introducing the use of the Universal Protocol will inevitably uncover errors. That is the exact point of the checklist.

The Universal Protocol's process, therefore, brings surgeons into direct contact with their own fallibility—an aspect of their humanness that they often fight to keep at bay. The brilliance of the Universal Protocol is that it uncovers errors in a manner that allows face-saving for every member of the surgical and procedural teams. By design, it provides the opportunity for minor human errors to be caught and addressed before they have an opportunity to contribute to devastating off-the-mark procedures. Because the checklist relies on a highly structured group process, it reinforces team effort and goes a long way toward overcoming the natural tendency to ascribe blame to a single person while also maintaining the surgeon's status as the team leader. In so doing, the Universal Protocol serves as a powerful reminder that lots of little things go wrong before a big mistake happens. It makes explicit the steps that must be taken to avoid catastrophe and establishes the surgeon alone is not responsible for preventing off-the-mark procedures.

Gawande told National Public Radio that when he first brought the Universal Protocol to surgeons for their use in the operating room, the predominant response was, "This is a waste of my time, I don't think it makes any difference."[24] Of those Gawande was able to convince to give it a try, 80 percent did not want to give it up. Another 20 percent remained dead set against using it even though 93 percent of the latter group indicated that they would want it used if they were undergoing surgery![25]

OVERCOMING RESISTANCE

Despite its simplicity and the proven effectiveness of this behavioral tool, it has not been universally implemented in US hospitals and surgical centers[26] or outpatient settings where invasive procedures are performed. Even in hospitals where use of the checklist has been adopted as policy, many physicians continue to resist using it or use it inappropriately. The resistance to its proper use is strong, as exemplified from this excerpt from *The Checklist Manifesto*:

> We doctors remain a long way from actually embracing the idea. The
> checklist has arrived in our operating rooms mostly from the outside

in and from the top down. It has come from finger-wagging health officials, who are regarded by surgeons as more or less the enemy, or from jug-eared hospital safety officers, who are about as beloved as the playground safety patrol. Sometimes it is the chief of surgery who brings it in, which means we complain under our breath rather than raise a holy tirade. But it is regarded as an irritation, as interference on our terrain. This is my patient. This is my operating room. And the way I carry out an operation is my business and my responsibility. So who do these people think they are, telling me what to do?[27]

In 2010, Gawande shared with National Public Radio listeners that he himself did not adopt it right away. After having convinced eight US hospitals to use the Universal Protocol and observe its value, he said he felt like a hypocrite for not using it. When he finally started using it, Gawande found the Universal Protocol "massively" improved the safety of his surgeries, noting, "I have not gotten through a week of surgery where the checklist has not caught a problem."[28]

While consulting with a hospital system that had (in theory) adopted the use of the Universal Protocol, I encountered a group of orthopedic surgeons who had experienced at least nine off-the-mark operations within a year. It quickly became evident that they—just like the physicians at Rhode Island Hospital where the three wrong-side brain surgeries occurred in a single year—had not incorporated the Universal Protocol into their workflow even though the hospital had adopted it as part of its policy. (As the saying goes, culture trumps policy.) After much pushback, a key hospital administrator settled on having orthopedic surgeons adopt parts of the Universal Protocol while allowing them to skip some steps associated with the first two time-outs before their patients were anesthetized. Not wanting to lose their business to another hospital in the area, the administrator caved to the surgeons' complaint that strict adherence would require them to redesign their workflow and would cost them time and money.

At the time, I was apoplectic with frustration. Later, I would learn that Gawande—perhaps the most prominent champion of the Universal Protocol—had discouraged hospitals from mandating obstinate surgeons from using the checklist or using it as it was designed. Gawande reasoned—correctly, I believe—that a backlash could form under a "forced regime." A single surgeon with a soured attitude could disparage the checklist and discourage others from trying it or using it appropriately.[29] While this might have been the best response when the Universal Protocol was a new checklist and in the early stages of implementation and testing, it is hard to imagine that informed patients would be equally tolerant today. Nonetheless, the manner in which the checklist becomes *universally* adopted is critical to its success.

Think again about the three wrong-brain surgeries within the span of a year happening at an Ivy League teaching hospital. With the benefit of hindsight, it became clear that surgeon buy-in about the hospital's Universal Protocol policy was lacking, and that this contributed to surgeons not using (or properly adhering to) the protocol. And as we know now, personnel outside the operating room had not been educated about the importance of getting things right before scheduling patients or sending patients to the operating room. To elicit full compliance will always require some modification of a hospital's broader-care delivery system.

Knowing that any surgical team is capable of committing an off-the-mark procedure and that the Universal Protocol is a powerful, efficient, and an essentially cost-free error prevention tool, it is hard to continue to excuse surgeons and other healthcare providers from using it. (Anecdotally, I am happy to report that the hospital where I recently underwent orthopedic surgery used the Universal Protocol in its entirety. Furthermore, it had incorporated the essential steps into information displayed on whiteboards on the wall in every patient's preop area. And the information was easy for everyone to see, including the steps that have been completed or still need to be completed.)

So, what can be done to ensure that the Universal Protocol is universally adopted in all hospitals and that referring clinics prepare patients to actively participate in the process? You can probably guess that generating interest in its use from the ground up is going to be the key to success. When healthcare providers begin to encounter patients who are sufficiently informed to request the Universal Protocol as part of their surgical or invasive care, they will shift from viewing its use as something forced on them from the-powers-that-be to considering it a choice they are willing to make to protect their business and their patients.

MAKING SURE THE "STUPID STUFF" ISN'T MISSED

The main purpose of the Universal Protocol is to eliminate off-the-mark procedures. However, this power-packed checklist also contains steps to ensure that potentially life-threatening details are not overlooked. During the preincision time-out, the checklist forces the surgical team to determine whether the correct and essential blood products, implants, devices, and special equipment are available before the first cut—the very things that could have made a difference in cases already discussed. While some have claimed that the Universal Protocol will not eliminate every single off-the-mark procedure, there is evidence that it can eliminate at least 73 to 75 percent of them.[30] If referring clinics were to be included in implementation processes, success would probably be higher (perhaps close to 100 percent) because over 10 percent of off-the-mark procedures are due to the surgical facility receiving incomplete or inaccurate information from referring medical offices.[31] Furthermore, there has been haphazard implementation of the checklist, lack of proper education regarding its use, and ongoing tolerance of an operating room culture with "tribal" affiliations between team members with clashing priorities.[32]

Even surgeons, who believe the tool is unnecessary, agree it is nearly impossible to argue that its use could be harmful. Once patients begin to understand the power and protection offered by consistent and proper use of the Universal Protocol, they—just like nearly all surgeons who used it—would want it to be used as part of their care.

Really, who can deny that modern medical care has become so complicated and fractured that it is simply not safe to perform an invasive procedure, including surgery, without conducting a preprocedure checklist? As surgeons and patients come to appreciate that the Universal Protocol is a checklist that is designed to make sure the "stupid stuff" isn't overlooked while clinicians are focused on complex clinical decisions, we will be well on our way toward widespread adoption of this powerful tool.

GREATER EXPECTATIONS

The public gasps when they hear the occasional news stories about horrific off-the-mark procedures, like those experienced by Willie King,

Susan Buchweiz, Baby Jessica, and Jésica Santillán. And rightfully so. Since the average person experiences seven surgeries in his lifetime, we all have skin in this game of getting things right. When the day arrives for your surgery or otherwise invasive procedure, you—like surgeons—are likely to be concerned about a lot of things (or overfocused on a few big things to the exclusion of some little things).

Nonetheless, as a patient, you have the greatest opportunity to protect against an off-the-mark procedure[33]; most of us just don't know it. That is why widespread understanding of the importance of the Universal Protocol, including performing preprocedure time-outs with patients' active involvement, must become the established routine. We need to get to the point where beginning the procedure without these vital pauses will come to feel as awkward as driving a car without a seatbelt now feels to most Americans. But everyone—not just surgeons—needs a structured process to make sure the "stupid stuff" isn't overlooked. Once you are wheeled into the operating room or procedural room, your ability to impact what transpires is limited. That is why there must be a "hard stop" to prevent the procedure from beginning without the third and last time-out.

In *The Checklist Manifesto*, Gawande recounts a clever "hard stop" method a surgeon devised for making sure he remembered to perform the third and final time-out of the Universal Protocol. The surgeon designed a metallic tent that was six inches long—just long enough to cover a scalpel—that was stenciled with the phrase "Cleared for Takeoff." He arranged for the tent to be placed in the surgical instruments kit. He instructed nurses to set the tent over the scalpel while laying out the instruments to be used in each surgery. This served as a cue—the sort of reminder that we all need—to run through the preincision time-out before the first cut. Furthermore, it also established that the surgeon could not begin the operation before the nurse gave her okay by removing the Cleared for Takeoff tent.

As you will read in chapter 6, what Gawande stumbled upon was a good example of a solution that had been "invisible in plain sight."

SEIZE THE DAY!

Compared to Semmelweis's fate for championing change, Gawande's has been golden. As described in chapter 3, Semmelweis, a surgeon in the early 1800s, was one of the first to proclaim that handwashing could eliminate the infections that were killing mothers who delivered their babies in Vienna hospitals. Semmelweis turned out to be correct, but his contemporaries never accepted his view. Rather, they declared him a lunatic, drove him out of town, and forced him into an insane asylum where he died from an infection. Fortunately for all of us, Dr. Gawande's peers have heralded him as an accomplished surgeon, a superb writer, and an internationally renowned medical innovator.

Carpe diem! Let's seize the day by putting Dr. Gawande's checklist manifesto into proper practice across the country and throughout the world. Let's make *universal* use of the Universal Protocol.

TAKING IT TO THE STREETS

Dr. Gawande's work and leadership on checklists has set the stage for engaging surgeons in the use of the Universal Protocol. Just as it is true for the prevention of healthcare-associated infections and deadly medical errors, patients will need to become informed and active participants in efforts to promote consistent use of the Universal Protocol.

In order to be able to confirm the correct procedure, physicians must learn to communicate clearly with patients about the name and nature of the planned procedure, and patients must learn the proper name of the procedure and what it involves. The days of passive patients who put blind trust in their physicians must come to a close. Patient passivity may never have been in the best interest of patients, but it most definitely is not a safe approach in today's complex, complicated, and fragmented healthcare system.

The tables below contain information that could be used to design educational campaigns and public alerts with corresponding sticky messages and sample language for communicating to prevent off-the-mark procedures. While it may not be advisable to adapt the Universal Protocol apart from systematic testing, the manner in which its material is communicated to the public can be adapted to meet a given hospital's or community's needs and preferences—a point discussed further in chapter 6.

Table 4.2.

WHAT YOU NEED TO KNOW
Off-the-Mark Procedures

Information for Patients

Each year thousands of surgeries and other invasive procedures are performed that involve the wrong patient, wrong body part, wrong place on a body part, or wrong procedure. These are called off-the-mark procedures (or wrong-site surgeries). When scheduling and performing surgery and other invasive procedures, minor errors can lead to major disasters.

To prevent common mix-ups, you must know the name of the procedure and exactly where the procedure will be performed on your body. On the day of the surgery, the healthcare provider who is going to operate will speak with you before you are sedated. Together with you, that provider will verify your identity, the name of the procedure, and where it is to be performed. The provider will mark your body in the right place. If any of these steps are overlooked, it is important to speak up before you are sedated.

Before allowing anyone to sedate you, make sure the provider who will be treating you takes a time-out to review your name and date of birth, the procedure you are to have, and marks your body accordingly. Speaking up for safety is not about challenging providers; it is about helping them. By participating in this process, you can help prevent tragic mishaps.

Information for Providers

When performing surgery and other invasive procedures, minor mix-ups are easily made, and such errors can have disastrous consequences. Therefore, the Joint Commission now requires use of the Universal Protocol to prevent off-the-mark procedures (also called wrong-site surgeries).

Through meticulous testing and revision, the Universal Protocol has emerged as an efficient and effective checklist that has the capacity to eliminate most, if not all, off-the-mark procedures. The beauty of the Universal Protocol is its balanced brevity and effectiveness. In addition to preventing off-the-mark procedures, the Universal Protocol ensures relevant documentation is present, diagnostic and radiology tests results are labeled and properly displayed, and any required blood products, implants, devices, and special equipment are available. The two to three-minute process required to complete the Universal Protocol also builds cohesion among team members, which increases the likelihood that someone will speak up for safety if necessary.

The Joint Commission now requires use of the Universal Protocol; however, it is your responsibility to use it consistently and in the manner that it was intended. Using a checklist is not an expression of weakness; it demonstrates your commitment to delivering the best care possible. Even highly competent surgeons and world-renown facilities have found the Universal Protocol frequently catches minor errors that could have led to tragic mistakes. After trying it, almost all surgeons say they would want the Universal Protocol used if they were to undergo surgery. Yet too many still resist using it (or resist using it properly) due to their denial of human and system fallibility. Don't be in denial.

Table 4.3.

PATIENT ACTION PLAN Off-the-Mark Procedures		
TIMING	**ACTION**	**✓**
Before scheduling a surgery or other invasive procedure	I know what an "off-the-mark procedure" is.	
	I understand that minor scheduling and preoperative mix-ups can lead to serious problems.	
	I am aware that even the best healthcare facilities and most competent providers sometimes make errors that can lead to major mistakes.	
	I know the name of my surgery or procedure and where it will be performed on my body.	
	I reviewed the Universal Protocol handout the clinic gave me, or I have considered reviewing the protocol online.	
When scheduling a surgery or other invasive procedure	I made sure the office confirmed: ☐ my name ☐ date of birth ☐ name of my procedure ☐ where the procedure will be performed on my body.	
	I asked what lab tests or radiographic images the facility needs and who is responsible for getting them there.	
	I asked if the Universal Protocol would be used with me.	
Before the day of the surgery or other invasive procedure	I practiced what to say if a time-out is not taken with me to confirm three important steps: 1. confirm my identity 2. review the name or location of my procedure, or 3. mark my body with the provider's initials.	
	I have considered having someone with me on the day of the procedure who can assist with this patient action plan.	
On the day of the surgery or invasive procedure	Before I am sedated, I will make sure my provider: ☐ verifies my identity ☐ reviews the name and location of my procedure ☐ marks my body on the correct spot with his or her initials	
	I will speak up if anything is incorrect, doesn't seem right, or if any of the three steps are skipped.	

Table 4.4.

WHAT YOU CAN SAY	
Sticky Message: **Catching Minor Mix-Ups Prevents Major Screw-Ups**	
When Scheduling a Surgery or an Invasive Procedure	
Patient Request	**Professional Response**
"Since we don't want anything to go wrong, do you use the Universal Protocol to perform time-outs with patients?"	"Yes, we use the Universal Protocol. Thank you for asking. I'm glad you know about it. It is important to participate in the time-outs, so you must learn the name of your procedure and know exactly where it will be performed on your body. We will write this out for you, but let's go over that information now. The name of your procedure is ___. It will be performed here ___. To make sure I've been clear, would you repeat that back to me?"
Before the Body Is Marked or Before the Patient Is Sedated	
Patient Request	**Professional Response**
"I'm glad you're marking my knee, but let's make sure I'm scheduled for the correct procedure."	"Absolutely! I almost marked your leg without verifying your ID and the name of your procedure. Let's start again."
"Wait, before you sedate me, the surgeon has not marked my body with her initials."	"Thank you for stopping me. I thought that had been done. I'll be back after the surgeon has reviewed the procedure with you and marked your body."
If you are interested in more detail, ask your healthcare providers for a copy of the Universal Protocol or search it online to (a) reinforce your familiarity with the checklist process and (b) support their efforts to consistently use the Universal Protocol.	

CHAPTER 5

Deadly Doses and Dangerous Drugs
Avoid Medication Errors and the Overuse of Opiates

Josie King

Eighteen-month-old Josie King was admitted to the hospital for second-degree burns. Over the course of about two weeks, Josie was treated with opiates to control her pain. When Josie's mother, Sorrel, arrived at the hospital early one morning, she found Josie to be unresponsive and called for help. The staff immediately gave Josie a dose of naloxone—a rescue medication that quickly and temporarily reverses the effect of opioids. The naloxone worked briefly, but a second dose was necessary. Both times Josie received the rescue medication, she perked up and wanted something to drink. Later that morning, Sorrel told Josie's surgeon, with whom she had developed a good relationship, what happened. The surgeon agreed to discontinue the painkillers and issued a verbal order to do so. A few hours later, while Sorrel was rubbing ointment on Josie's feet, a gruff nurse who was new to Josie and Sorrel arrived with a syringe of the pain medication in hand. Sorrel questioned the nurse, but the nurse rebuffed her concerns. The nurse injected the opiate in Josie and almost immediately Josie's eyes rolled back in her head. She quickly became unresponsive. Sorrel screamed for help, but it was too late. Josie went into cardiac arrest and experienced oxygen deprivation that left her brain dead. As a result, two days before she was to be discharged from the hospital, Josie died.[1]

NOTHING ABOUT ME WITHOUT ME

Even though a great deal has been written about this event, including *Josie's* Story, a memoir by Sorrel King, it still has great currency for bringing to light issues related to the safe use of drugs inside (and outside) hospitals and other healthcare settings.[2] The cascade of errors that led to Josie's death is what makes it such an illustrative, though heartbreaking, patient safety story. How the hospital responded to Josie's death is as inspiring as the story is tragic.

During the course of being treated for second-degree burns, doctors had placed a central line catheter in Josie. The central line was used to make it easier to administer essential fluids and medications. Along the way, the line became infected. Because Josie's doctors planned to discharge her within two days, they decided to remove the central line and administer medications orally. As a side effect to the oral antibiotics, Josie began having diarrhea and vomiting. Without a central line in place to deliver fluids, Josie became dehydrated. When a patient becomes dehydrated, his or her condition can deteriorate rapidly, which, in turn, can cause the body to go into a dangerous state of septic shock. Sometimes behavioral signs of septic shock are apparent before clinical tests and other metrics make the problem obvious. Indeed, Josie's fluid input and output metrics looked okay, but they belied what Josie's mother saw. As you will learn, Sorrel's observations and resultant concern were mostly ignored. Consider this excerpt from Sorrel's book:

> I asked her [the nurse] what she was doing and told her that Dr. Paidas had given orders for Josie not to receive more methadone.
> "Don't give it to her," I said as she neared Josie's bed.
> "The orders have been changed," she responded.
> Something didn't seem right. Why were the orders changed? Should I knock the drug out of her hands and scream for help? Was I missing something? Stop, slow down, I told myself. I am at Johns Hopkins, the best hospital in the country. These doctors and nurses are the smartest. They know more than I do. They must have changed the orders for a reason, a good reason. They know what they are doing. I moved aside and stood there as Brenda [the nurse] squirted the drug into Josie's mouth. I continued rubbing ointment on her feet.
> "Look, a crocodile tear," Amy [another nurse who was familiar with Josie] said.
> I looked and there it was, one single tear sliding down Josie's cheek. I wiped it away, thinking to myself how strange it was that in the two weeks

since Josie and I had been in the hospital this was the very first tear I had seen. I began taking off my gloves and cleaning up, but when I looked back at Josie I stopped dead in my tracks. Her eyes had rolled back in her head. "Josie? Josie!" I shook her. She was not responding. I screamed for help. Amy screamed for help and starting pushing buttons on the monitors.

"Look at her! Look at her! Someone help!" I screamed.

A dozen nurses and doctors raced to her bed with metal tables and trays and equipment. I felt myself being led out of the room and into the hall . . . They put me in a small, windowless room. A chaplain stood quietly in the corner, and I wondered why he was there.[3]

At first, the hospital told Josie's parents they suspected Josie had succumbed to a massive infection, but Sorrel thought otherwise. Eventually, the hospital realized that the opioid painkiller (methadone) was central to this event. Josie's body did not tolerate the last shot of methadone. After the drug was administered, Josie experienced a cardiac arrest that led to oxygen deprivation. Because Josie no longer had a central line, it was difficult to get rescue medications into her quickly. The time without oxygen resulted in brain damage. And Josie, who was on the verge of being discharged after more than two weeks of successful hospital care, died.

The surgeon ordered pain medications stopped because Josie no longer appeared to be in pain and because opioids can cause or intensify dehydration, which had become apparent to Josie's mother. However, the pain management specialist, an anesthesiologist who saw Josie later that morning, was more concerned about the consequences of abrupt withdrawal from the opioids. By the time the anesthesiologist saw Josie, the surgeon had left the unit, although one of his surgical residents was still there. The resident disagreed with the anesthesiologist's concern, so the anesthesiologist pulled rank. Without speaking to the surgeon, she ordered more opioids (although at a lower dose).

What makes this case disturbing is that the anesthesiologist knew Sorrel had her guard up against more pain medication for her infant daughter, yet she chose not to share her thoughts or decision about ordering more painkillers with Sorrel—effectively cutting the patient's advocate out of the loop. When Sorrel objected to the nurse giving the medication, the nurse dismissed her concerns and disregarded her objection.

The Swiss cheese effect had taken hold. A cascade of errors culminated in failure of the worst kind. The hospital didn't protect Josie
from picking up an infection, a communication breakdown between
physicians led to poor management of a powerful painkiller, a failure to
communicate prevented a mother from having a say in her child's care,
and a nurse disregarded a mother's expressed objection to treatment.
Oops, oops, oops, oops, boom!

Josie's story screams for better teamwork to improve communication among all members of the healthcare team. Patients and families
should not have to bully their way onto the team. After Josie's death,
many hospitals started completing rounds at the patients' bedsides,
with the express purpose of involving them and their families in the
decision-making process. There is ample evidence to demonstrate that
this type of communication improves the quality and safety of care.[4]
Bedside rounding has been shown to add additional and relevant information in nearly half (46 percent) of the rounds.[5] Regardless, rounding at the bedside supports the humane and compassionate concept of
"nothing about me, without me"—something that has been discussed
by patient safety leaders for some time[6] and that the National Patient
Safety Foundation aspires to enable all patients to express.[7] After all,
a physician's propensity to err is great, although often denied, and a
patient is often the only person who can provide a critical piece of information that may avert disaster.

A MEDICATED SOCIETY

Modern societies, and the United States in particular, have become re-
flexive in associating symptoms with drug interventions. At last count,
seven out of ten Americans take at least one prescription medication
on a daily basis. More than half of all Americans take two types of
daily prescriptions, and nearly a quarter takes five or more daily.[8] In
one year alone (2011), 4.02 billion drug prescriptions were written for
US patients. This equates to an average of thirteen prescriptions for
every man, woman, and child, with roughly one new prescription every
month for every American.[9] This massive amount of daily drug use
does not include over-the-counter or hospital-administered drugs. Research indicates that over 80 percent of US adults use over-the-counter

drugs as a first response to minor ailments with a total of 2.9 billion retail trips annually to purchase over-the-counter medications.[10]

Perhaps it should be no surprise that dangerous drug combinations represent a leading cause of hospitalization. National data indicate that by 2005, nearly 7 percent of all US hospital admissions were specifically for adverse drug reactions,[11] with a rate that is more than one-and-one-half times higher among elderly patients.[12] In addition to the medications patients are on when they are admitted to a hospital, additional drugs are almost always added to their regimen after they are admitted. Ensuring that hospital patients receive the right medications, at the right times, in the right doses, and through the right routes can be extremely complex and complicated.

EPIC-LEVEL DRUG HARM

Like healthcare-associated infections, hospital-induced medication errors have reached epidemic proportions. They alone represent a major public health crisis that appears to be intensifying each year. Fifteen years ago, *To Err Is Human* estimated that seven thousand US hospital patients were dying annually as a result of medication errors. It is now widely accepted that this figure represents a significant underestimate of the magnitude of the problem, then and now. Besides the historic issue of the underreporting of hospital-based medication errors, the number of medications that patients take before, during, and after they are hospitalized is much greater today than it was in previous decades. With the increased rate of medication use, the risk of medication-related harm and error has increased exponentially.

Looking at data from a single year (2011), 286.2 million drug orders were placed for patients admitted to US emergency departments, and another 329.2 million orders were placed for patients admitted to US hospital outpatient departments, totaling over 615 million drug orders among patients treated at hospitals without being admitted.[13] In that same year, millions more drug orders were placed for patients who were admitted to inpatient units.

A major investigation of data during the 2006 to 2008 time frame indicated that more than seventeen billion drug orders were written for hospitalized patients annually.[14] Also in a single year (2000), individuals living in nursing homes were found to receive an average of nearly seven routine prescription medications per day and between two and three additional medications on an "as needed basis."[15] And the rate of prescription drug use among nursing home residents has been on the rise ever since.[16]

It is impossible to come up with a single figure or estimate that would accurately capture the extent of harm that results from current rates of drug ordering, prescribing, and over-the-counter purchasing. That is a black number—a number that is not precisely knowable. Nonetheless, the US Food and Drug Administration has a reporting system that sheds some light on the subject. This system, which is commonly called MedWatch, is the world's largest database of voluntary, spontaneous reports of adverse drug reactions and drug errors.

An *adverse reaction* refers to instances of unintended or harmful drug reactions that could not be predicted, such as a first-time allergic reaction. A *drug error* refers to a preventable mistake that has the potential to cause harm while in the control of a healthcare professional, patient, or consumer. For example, prescribing a drug to which a patient has a known allergy would count as a drug error.

While MedWatch includes all adverse drug events, the voluntary nature of the system assures that its data generates gross underestimates of the full magnitude of adverse drug events, including an underreporting of drug errors.

A few years ago, researchers used MedWatch to conduct an in-depth analysis of adverse drug reactions from 1998 (when the system was first created) through 2005.[17] They discovered that both the rate of US prescriptions and adverse drug reactions increased each year. In 2005 (the last year of the study), MedWatch documented 15,107 fatal adverse drug reaction cases and another 89,842 serious adverse drug reaction cases—cases that caused harm but did not result in death. Furthermore, the annual increase in adverse events grew four times faster than the rate of prescriptions, especially among elderly patients.

FREQUENCY AND COST OF DRUG ERRORS IN HOSPITALS

To get a handle on the relative frequency of adverse reactions versus drug errors, one study looked at ten common types of unanticipated patient harm and then checked to see how often each harm category was due to an unavoidable complication versus an error. Only one out of the ten categories was more likely to occur as a result of an unavoidable complication—drug-related events. Specifically, error was involved in only 10 percent of drug-related instances of harm. Yet in the other nine categories of patient harm, human error was involved in 35 percent to 91 percent of the cases.[18] Even a 10 percent error rate among the high volume of hospital drug orders would amount to tens of millions of medication errors per year, a significant portion of which would result in death or serious harm. In fact, that is precisely what more recent evidence suggests. A 2013 publication that was based on a rigorous analysis of national databases indicated that, as of 2008, over 1.7 billion drug orders were processed in US hospitals with up to 1.7 million drug errors.

To Err Is Human suggested that—based on a conservative assessment—seven thousand medication-related hospitals deaths occurred among US patients each year.[19] At the time (1999), this figure was shocking. Today, patient safety experts can only wish that the magnitude of harm were as low as that report originally estimated.

Recently, the Institute of Medicine estimated approximately one medication error occurs per day for every US hospital patient.[20] Some researchers have documented that at least one million serious hospital medication errors occur each year;[21] others have estimated that approximately 20 percent of hospital medication errors could be life threatening.[22] Astounding as such figures are, recent research by the Office of the Inspector General indicates that the rate of preventable drug harm to Medicare beneficiaries in nursing homes exceeds that of hospitals.[23]

No matter how you look at it, the rate of medication error and associated harm that occur in hospitals, nursing homes, and the community is beyond any rational level of comfort. And this is an expensive problem. As of ten years ago, on average, medication errors added $2,000 to the cost of a hospitalization, which amounted to over $7.5 billion in annual US hospital charges.[24] In today's dollars that would amount to over $11 billion annually.

WHY SO MANY ERRORS?

How could there *not* be so many medication errors? Within a hospital environment, it is common for one physician to order a medication that one or multiple nurses will administer, while other physicians and nurses monitor its effects and alter the patient's subsequent drug regimen. Along the way, the prescribing physician must communicate the treatment plan with whomever might administer the medication. Once a drug is ordered, it must be obtained from the pharmacy, checked against the patient record for allergies or other adverse indications of its use, and administered to the right patient, in the right dose, via the right route, and at the right time. At every step, someone must determine, through observation or inquiry, whether the medication is working as intended and without ill effect. Every step of this process must be documented, and every step is a source of potential error.

Patients on adult inpatient medicine units will typically receive medications for several different chronic and acute conditions. Such patients could easily receive fifteen or twenty individual doses of medication administered by three or more different nurses in a single twenty-four-hour period.[25]

Research suggests that serious drug errors are about as likely to occur when ordered and administered, although they are less likely to occur during the transcription phase.[26] Ordering errors often result from insufficient knowledge on the part of providers with prescription privileges—a factor over which patients have essentially no control once they are hospitalized. Patients also have little or no control over errors that are made by a clerk during the process of transcribing a provider's order or during the process of medications being dispensed to a hospital unit. However, patients can be enormously helpful in eliminating errors during the administration process.

Medication administration errors tend to occur for one of two reasons: first, "silly" and "stupid" mistakes that any of us can make (akin to pouring orange juice in our morning coffee or on our cereal); second, communication breakdowns. Regarding the first common cause: minds are prone to frequent slips and lapses, especially if we are distracted, tired, stressed, or mentally overloaded—the very conditions with which nurses must contend on a daily basis. As summarized in the table below, there are few common sorts of mistakes and factors that contribute to medication administration errors.[27]

Table 5.1.

Common Sources of Medication Error	
Simple Miscalculations	Basic mathematical calculation errors can result in drug errors through careless transposing of units. For example, confusing micrograms and milligrams would result in a patient receiving one thousand times the intended dose of a drug. Misplacing or misreading decimal placements leads to similar types of dosage errors.
Look-Alike, Sound-Alike Drugs	It is easy to confuse drugs with names that look or sound similar to each other. For example, Losec (that treats heartburn, stomach ulcers, and gastroesophageal reflux disease) is known to get confused with Lasix (that treats fluid retention and high blood pressure).
Illegible Handwriting	The problem of poor handwriting is so great that the Joint Commission alerted hospitals and healthcare professionals to the fact that prescriber handwriting is implicated in many drug errors.
Verbal Orders	Verbal orders—regardless of whether they are shared in person or by phone—are more prone to error than handwritten orders. Different accents, dialects, and pronunciations as well as background noise, interruptions, and unfamiliar drug names and terminology often create problems when hearing and interpreting verbal orders. For example, it would be easy to mishear an order for erythromycin instead of azithromycin; an order for Klonopin 0.1 mg instead of clonidine 0.1 mg; or an order for Viscertol rather than Vistaril.

When walking into an unfamiliar unit, juggling a handful of sick patients, or trying to complete all the necessary tasks at the end of a shift, it's all too easy for anybody to experience a degree of mental overload. To combat information overload, our brains search and sweep the environment until something grabs its attention, and it masterfully fills in the gaps when information is missing. Without realizing it, we direct our attention to what seems like the most salient pieces of information and blot the rest out of our conscious minds. Thus, we routinely act upon a picture that is based on "just a flickering view" of reality. The result is called *inattentional blindness*—instances when the eyes see what the mind expects rather than what is really there.[28]

TECHNOLOGY TO THE RESCUE—YES! (AND NO!)

Because medication errors are so numerous and a leading cause of healthcare-induced harm,[29] the industry has expended considerable effort and resources to develop health information technology (IT) specific to reducing this problem. Three leading health IT interventions include computerized physician order entry (CPOE) systems, barcode medication administration (BCMA) systems, and electronic medical administration record (eMAR) systems.

Computerized physician order entry (CPOE) systems are electronic prescribing systems that intercept errors when they most commonly occur—at the time medications are ordered. With CPOE, physicians enter orders into a computer rather than on paper. Orders are integrated with patient information, including laboratory and prescription data. The order is then automatically checked for potential errors or problems. Specific benefits of CPOE include prompts that warn against the possibility of drug interaction, allergy, or overdose; accurate, current information that helps physicians keep up with new drugs as they are introduced into the market; drug-specific information that eliminates confusion among drug names that sound alike; improved communication between physicians and pharmacists; and reduced healthcare costs due to improved efficiency.[30]

Recognizing that CPOE systems have a remarkable potential to reduce the rate of error, national healthcare organizations support Leapfrog's ongoing efforts to drive more hospitals to safely implement and use them. Each year, the number of hospitals using CPOE continues to rise, but "it's troubling that not all CPOE systems give appropriate warnings for orders that might have tragic consequences for patients."[31] In order to fully meet Leapfrog's current standards, hospitals must adopt CPOE for at least 75 percent of their medication orders using a CPOE system that includes provider-error prevention strategies and demonstrate their inpatient system can alert physicians to at least half of common, serious prescribing errors. They demonstrate the safety of their systems through a simulation process that has them run mock orders provided by Leapfrog through their systems to see how many known errors their system flags.

The 2014 Leapfrog Hospital Survey results indicated that 34 percent of US hospitals voluntarily completed the annual survey and that over 90 percent of them used CPOE in at least one hospital unit. Fifty-nine percent of Leapfrog-reporting hospitals entered at least 75 percent of their orders electronically. During the testing of the effectiveness of systems used in hospitals that completed the Leapfrog simulation, it was discovered that failure rates remain unacceptably high. During simulation tests, CPOE systems failed to issue a warning on potentially harmful medication orders 36 percent of the time. Further, the number of potentially fatal orders that weren't flagged by CPOE systems remained above 10 percent, at 13.9 percent.[32]

Like CPOE, barcode technology has also been useful in reducing, though not eliminating, errors during the drug-dispensing and administration phases.

Barcode medication administration (BCMA) systems are electronic scanning systems that intercept medication errors at the point of administration. When administering medications with BCMA, a nurse scans a barcode on the patient's wristband to confirm that the patient is the right patient. The nurse then scans a barcode on the medicine to verify that it is the right medication at the right dose, given at the right time by the right route. BCMA is typically used in conjunction with electronic medication administration record (eMAR) systems. An eMAR serves as the communication interface that automatically documents the administration of medication into certified Electronic Health Record (EHR) technology. By linking BCMA with the eMAR, information on medication administration is captured in a much timelier manner than a manual documentation process can accomplish.[33]

Each of these technological advances—CPOE, eMAR, and BCMA—has the capacity to reduce drug errors in every phase of the process, from ordering to administering medications. Rates of error have been reported for each phase of the hospital medication process. Maximal benefit can be realized by using health information technology systems in a coordinated fashion. For example, both eMAR and BCMA can eliminate some medication errors, but using these two systems together increases the capacity to eliminate error. And although routinely using barcodes has proved to be useful in healthcare, they are still only used in about 65 percent of US hospitals. Forthcoming Leapfrog standards will help address BCMA gaps and drive remaining hospitals to implement BCMA and help all hospitals to use BCMA safely.

Table 5.2.

Using Technology to Reduce Drug Errors in Hospitals			
Medication Process	**Percentage of Errors**	**Technology**	**Potential to Avert Errors**
Ordering	39%	CPOE	55%
Dispensing	11%	BCMA	67%
Administering	38%	BCMA + eMAR	51%

Another 12% of errors are estimated to occur when a clerk transcribes a physician order, which CPOE has the potential to eliminate. All figures are based on several independent studies presented to the Center for Medication Safety Advancement in October 2012.

Technology is important, but technology alone cannot solve the problem of medication errors; it is never foolproof. Technology is only as good as the systems that support it and the people who use it. Some spectacular CPOE implementation failures forced the industry to accept that CPOE systems are not "plug and play" systems. Since CPOE systems were first introduced, healthcare has learned a lot more about how these systems affect workflow and how to prepare providers for their use. A growing number of hospitals hire outside consulting groups to assist them with training during system go-lives.[34] Because healthcare was willing to learn from early CPOE and other technology-related failures, it has improved patient safety.[35] But it is also fair to say that too many of the individuals using electronic health information systems on a routine basis remain unaware of inherent system shortcomings and associated risk factors, as exemplified by what happened to a Chicago couple and their newborn.[36]

Genesis Burkett

Genesis Burkett, a tiny infant, was born to first-time parents who had experienced two previous miscarriages. Although Genesis was born prematurely, he was expected to survive and do well. While being cared for in a neonatal intensive care unit, Genesis received what was supposed to be routine fluid therapy involving a saline solution. He was accidentally administered a dose that was sixty times higher than prescribed. He died soon after this incident. His death resulted from a series of errors that began with the kind of human error that people often make when filling out electronic forms. A pharmacy technician mistakenly typed the wrong information into a computer. Because of the mix-up, an automatic machine dispensed a fluid bag for an adult, ultimately resulting in a massive overdose of sodium chloride. This error was compounded by the fact that the IV mixing machine—that could have identified the problem—did not have the automatic alerts feature turned on. Furthermore, the IV bag's label did not match its contents and the pharmacist never double-checked the label. To make matters worse, blood tests showed that the baby's sodium levels were high, so a physician ordered a repeat test; however, a technician assumed the initial lab reading was wrong and the repeat test was never performed. A year after Genesis's parents filed a lawsuit, the hospital agreed to pay them an $8.25 million settlement.[37]

The Genesis Burkett tragedy showcases how easily information that is incorrectly entered into an electronic medical system—a decidedly human error—can be perpetuated throughout the delivery care process through the use of technology. It also highlights the dangers of overdependence on technology. In a public statement following the Genesis Burkett case, a spokesperson for the hospital where the event occurred appropriately said:

This event has only heightened our focus on patient care. We have taken comprehensive steps across [the healthcare system] to ensure this type of tragedy does not happen again. The steps include having pharmacists double-check IV bags, making sure that what is on an IV bag reflects what is actually in it.[38]

Thinking in terms of the Swiss Cheese Model described in chapter 2, the pharmacist made the initial error (human error) that led to the wrong medication being dispensed to the ward (technology-related error). However, once on the ward, the nurse failed to check the label on the medication against the order that was in the patient's medical record (human error). As noted above, other blunders occurred as well, including a decision not to have the relevant eMAR alert turned on (system issue). A simple slip or lapse of attention—the kind of error that everybody is prone to make on occasion—will sometimes initiate a cascade of errors and set the domino effect into motion. At the end of the day, safety is a people business, and the human factor can never be forgotten. Everyone must play his or her part to maintain safe care.

OVERCOMING A FALSE SECURITY

As it did for me, perhaps the Genesis Burkett tragedy will remind other behavioral scientists of the infamous Kitty Genovese case. Ms. Genovese was a young woman who was stabbed to death near her home in the Queens borough of New York City. The story made headline news because numerous neighbors witnessed the stabbing, but nobody did anything. While some of the details have been disputed over time, this horrific urban legend prompted many psychologists to study what is now recognized as the bystander apathy or bystander effect. The *bystander effect* refers to the reality that people are less likely to take action to protect someone when others are around who could also do so. The more bystanders, the more diffused an individual's sense of responsibility becomes and the less likely it is that anybody will offer help. In one experiment that recreated the Kitty Genovese case, 70 percent of people called out for help when they were alone with a woman in distress while only 40 percent did so when other people were around.[39]

The field of patient safety has its corollaries to the Kitty Genovese case. It is easy for individual members of the healthcare team to discount the importance of their safety precautions, believing that other known safeguards are in play. Technology is one of those other protective barriers notorious for lulling healthcare professionals into a false sense of security by diffusing the sense of individual responsibility. The existence of error-catching technology can reduce the likelihood that providers will engage in error-prevention safety practices because automated technology that rarely, if ever, gets something wrong minimizes our felt need to be vigilant. And when something doesn't seem right, we are prone to distrust our own perceptions. So the more contact with technology that alerts people to error, the more ingrained their false sense of security can become.

In a similar way, people sometimes discount their perceptions because of what psychologists refer to as *groupthink*. It occurs when a group of people becomes cohesive enough that a member of the group becomes reluctant to share contradictory information because he wants to maintain harmony. More succinctly, business writer Megan McArdle calls this *groupidity*: doing something stupid because other people around you seem to think it is safe.[40]

Nurses are especially vulnerable to this phenomenon because humans are more likely to take unsafe risks when working in teams or working under pressure—exactly how nurses routinely operate. But so too are more diverse groups of healthcare providers who work in teams and under intense circumstances—like ICU teams that are tight or surgical teams that have worked together for a long time. Unfortunately, the cohesion that helps teams to work together smoothly can also contribute to a sense of overconfidence and lead team members to engage in unacceptable levels of risk, collectively rationalizing away obvious warning signs.[41]

UNINTENDED CONSEQUENCES

With workloads that are already barely manageable, whenever a new procedure or policy is introduced, nurses will discover shortcuts to keep moving at their usual pace. When a shortcut is found to work well for one person, with barely a wink or a nod, others pick up the trick. The more people engage in these practices without them being questioned, the more ingrained they become until they are thought of as acceptable workarounds.

A *workaround* is a method, sometimes used temporarily, for achieving a task or goal when the usual or planned method isn't working. In information technology, a workaround is often used to overcome hardware, programming, or communication problems. Once a problem is fixed, a workaround is usually abandoned.[42]

For example, when barcoding is used properly, additional time is required to appropriately scan every medication dose and patient wristband at the patient's bedside. Because medication administration has been noted to occupy up to one-third of work time among hospital nurses,[43] it is a natural target for timesaving workarounds. One study documented fifteen types of barcoding workarounds. For example, when barcoding was introduced on hospital wards, nurses were observed affixing patient identification barcodes to computer carts, scanners, doorjambs, and their personal clothing and to carry several patients' prescanned medications on carts as they moved between patient rooms.[44] Some nurses were seen cutting the bands off patients' wrists to avoid needing to be with the patient when entering information into an eMAR system. For the same reason and to the same ill effect, when there aren't enough medication dispensing machines (cabinets that provide computer-controlled storage, dispensing, and tracking capabilities), nurses have been known to stockpile unused medications and "borrow" them to give to another patient when in a hurry. They also saved time by removing medications for multiple patients while the cabinet was open for only one patient and grabbing multiple doses at once.

On a system level, it can be difficult to distinguish a valuable adaptation from a misguided workaround. Once a CPOE system is implemented, hospitals adjust their capabilities, especially by turning off specific system alerts. Some alerts occur so frequently that they run the risk of *alert fatigue*, which is "caused by excessive numbers of warnings about items such as potentially dangerous drug interactions. As a result, providers may pay less attention to or even ignore some vital alerts, thus limiting these systems' effectiveness."[45] A review of seventeen studies found that, as of 2006, providers were overriding or ignoring 49 percent to 90 percent of CPOE alerts.[46]

While consulting with a healthcare system, a cardiologist convinced the hospital to turn off a commonly occurring drug-interaction alert. He reasoned that he and his colleagues, like all reasonably competent cardiologists, were keenly aware of the risks associated with the particular drug interaction and knew how to manage it safely. The problem was that physicians from other specialties weren't as aware of such risks or how to handle them, and physicians from the emergency department were using the same drugs with some regularity. After the alert was turned off, two serious safety events, including a death, occurred before the healthcare system realized it needed a broader and multidisciplinary CPOE modification review process.

As an organization that monitors the safety of CPOE systems post-implementation, Leapfrog has emerged as a leading advocate for establishing standards around leadership oversight and training before, during, and after implementation of new health information technology. Progress has been made in recent years, and it is expected to continue.

THE HUMAN SIDE OF DRUG SAFETY

The information presented so far should make it apparent just how hard it is to ensure patients receive the right medication and *only* the right medications. As Gawande explains in *The Checklist Manifesto*, some four thousand drugs now exist for treating over thirteen thousand diagnostic options, making the process of getting things right both a complex and complicated undertaking. Drug safety is complex because it is not always possible to know the best medications to prescribe. This requires thoughtful decision making that is based on a lot of information that a physician might not have at his or her fingertips or might not have learned. Drug safety is also a complicated process because it requires attention to many details and/or steps.

A person's ability to attend and focus, or what is sometimes referred to as a *state of mindfulness*, has a significant impact on the likelihood of error. Mindfulness is highly variable from one day to the next, and it can shift without a moment's notice. As noted earlier, nurses are chronically working under conditions that tax their ability to stay focused and concentrate, leaving a wealth of opportunity for error to occur during the medication administration process. So healthcare has developed the concept of the *Five Rights of Medication Administration* to help nurses cue themselves into being mentally cognizant of their actions when giving medications to patients. The Five Rights refer to the properties listed below.

1	2	3	4	5
Right	Right	Right	Right	Right
Patient	Drug	Dose	Route	Time

The Five Rights of Medication Administration can help catch many of the errors that commonly occur during the medication administration process. However, the Five Rights are intended to be the end goal of the medication process, not the be-all and end-all of medication safety. The Institute for Safe Medication Practices writes this about the Five Rights:

> They are merely broadly stated goals, or desired outcomes, of safe medication practices that offer no procedural guidance on how to achieve these goals. Thus, simply holding healthcare practitioners accountable for giving the right drug to the right patient in the right dose by the right route at the right time fails miserably to ensure medication safety. Adding a sixth, seventh, or eighth right (e.g., right reason, right drug formulation, right line attachment) is not the answer, either.[47]

The Five Rights focus on individual performance and not on human factors and system defects that may make completing the tasks difficult or impossible,[48] so the Institute for Safe Medication Practices also warns about the danger of engaging in workarounds, even when they don't result in bad outcomes:

> The healthcare practitioners' duty is not so much to achieve the five rights, but to follow the procedural rules designed by the organization to produce these outcomes. And if the procedural rules cannot be followed because of system issues, healthcare practitioners also have a duty to report the problem so it can be remedied.[49]

Of course, it is equally imperative that those with the authority to make the system changes respond when medication workarounds are identified. Otherwise, providers will continue to use them and place patients at risk. After all, most nurses carry intense workloads and employ workarounds because they seem like practical ways to get the job done—not because they intend to cause harm. When nobody listens to real challenges they face, nurses carry on in the best ways they know how—even if it means disregarding some safeguards.

NO MAGIC BULLET, BUT TWO GOOD HABITS

A patient can easily be caught in moments that exist between when workarounds surface and when they are eradicated through systemic hospital improvements. They are also vulnerable to receiving medications in moments when a nurse is distracted. There is no magic bullet to making sure that every patient receives the right medication and only the right medication. At the actual point of medication administration, there is, however, a strategy that can significantly reduce the chance of an error.

Whenever possible, patients and family members must partner with nurses to make sure that two essential medication safety habits occur: (1) verification of patient identification and (2) a review of our Five Rights. Just like handwashing and time-outs, the general public can learn when these two safety habits should occur and observe whether they do occur because they involve concrete and straightforward actions.

In chapter 4, I discussed the fallout from improper patient identification before surgeries and other invasive procedures, but the failure to properly identify patients during medical testing, transfusions, the discharging of newborns to families, and the administration of medications also causes problems. The World Health Organization, the Joint Commission, and the Joint Commission International came together to draft a solution to the patient identification problem. Jointly, they advise that, whenever possible, *proper patient identification* must: (a) actively involve patients in the identification process, (b) begin by asking patients to identify themselves by name, and (c) verify patient identity by at least two pieces of information—usually name and date of birth, which are to be checked against other documentation such as a medication order, medical record, or lab order.[50] Furthermore, an in-depth analysis of patient engagement efforts that included patient interviews reported that patients say they are more likely to speak up when providers introduce themselves before treating patients because they equate it with an invitation to participate.[51]

As noted above, technology can help avert patient safety mishaps by catching identification errors; however, technology will not eliminate the need for some degree of human checking. During a twenty-month period, 236 voluntary reports were made of wrong patient identification due to missing wristbands and wristbands with incorrect information.[52] Even as barcode technology improves, there will still be distinct advantages of verbal confirmation of a patient's identity. First, technology itself, and the energy source that supports it, can malfunction. Second, the identification process is an opportunity for a momentary patient-nurse interaction that can create a sense of caring—something that helps the healing process and has been corroded since the introduction of electronic health records systems and related technologies.

Asking patients to participate in a review of the Five Rights may seem too complicated, but it isn't. More importantly, to the extent that nurses embrace the "nothing about me without me" concept, it should seem unfathomable to administer drug therapy to patients without their participation in the Five Rights (whenever patient status allows). Too often, though, nurses walk into patient rooms and change their IV bags or say things like, "I'm just going to give you some medication now" and proceed to deliver medication through existing portals.

Including patients in the review of drugs they are to be given creates an opportunity for a two-person check. For certain, these would be imperfect, but independent double checks do reduce error substantially. The Institute for Safe Medication Practices reports that, time and again, use of independent double checks has been shown to catch up to 95 percent of errors.[53] Nonetheless, nurses and other healthcare providers have resisted routine use of independent double checks because it is incredibly time-consuming to track down another healthcare provider. They also object to heavy reliance on independent double checks because when the process becomes too routine, it is easy to perform it on autopilot—checking without really paying attention to what is written or communicated.

Having patients participate in the medication checking process does not suffer from either of the sources of resistance associated with independent double checks between two providers, while also conferring additional benefits. First, the amount of time it takes to include patients is miniscule compared to the time it takes to track down another provider. The second person—the patient—is always right there. Second, for patients, the process of double-checking medication will never become as automatic as it is for nurses who must do it every day of their working lives. Also, the patient typically has the greatest investment in getting things right, and the process itself can help patients see that they are part of the healthcare team.

When patients come to appreciate the importance of these concrete safety behaviors, they will become tolerant, if not outright appreciative, of what may seem to many like annoying and dimwitted redundancies. In the process and without realizing it, people will be acting their way into a new way of thinking about medication safety. Once people are tuned into the magnitude of medication errors and patients start collaborating with nurses on medication administration safety habits, word will spread about errors that were caught and near disasters that were averted. As these scenarios unfold and stories get told, the importance of verifying patient IDs and reviewing drug orders with patients will become understood and reinforced. This safety behavior will become accepted as "just what patients and nurses do."

THE SPECIAL CASE OF OPIATE PAINKILLERS

I thought about ending this chapter after discussing specific safety habits that can help eliminate medication administration errors. However, the United States is in the throes of a terrifying heroin epidemic that is related to the use of opiates in hospitals and freestanding surgical centers. The problem is seriously threatening the safety of individuals, hospitals, and society. According to the Centers for Disease Control and Prevention, 1.9 million Americans are struggling with addiction to opiate painkillers.

> Several factors are likely to have contributed to the severity of the current prescription drug abuse problem. They include drastic increases in the number of prescriptions written and dispensed, greater social acceptability for using medications for different purposes, and aggressive marketing by pharmaceutical companies. These factors together have helped create the broad "environmental availability" of prescription medications in general and opioid analgesics in particular . . . [which] account for the greatest proportion of the prescription drug abuse problem.[54]

The CDC further clarified that some people become addicted to opiates because they fail to take them as prescribed (taking more than the number of pills prescribed at any one time or taking them too frequently) or because they mix them with alcohol and other drugs. However, a small number of people may become addicted even when taking them as prescribed.

Drug addiction is a complex issue; so what does it have to do with patient safety? The answer: plenty. And if you were to ask Carolyn Weems that question, she would quickly make the connection clear. The strongest risk factor for heroin use is addiction to prescription painkillers—the very class of drugs that are prescribed for over half of American hospital patients. So, who is Carolyn Weems? She is a school board member in the city of Virginia Beach, Virginia—the area of the country where I live—and a mother who recently lost her twenty-one-year-old daughter, Caitlyn. Caitlyn was a much-loved soccer star that suffered a number of sports injuries that required surgery and other treatments. As Weems explains, Caitlyn would get injured, the family would seek treatment for the injuries, and Caitlyn would be prescribed pain medications.[55]

Recounting how the properties of pain medications and heroin are virtually identical, Weems refers to Caitlyn's prescription drugs—Percocet, Vicodin, Dilaudid, Fentanyl, Demerol, and Darvon—as heroin.[56] If you're like me, hearing this for the first time may sound alarmist, but Weems's perspective turns out to be accurate. Because prescription opiates are not cut with other substances that dealers use to make heroin easier and more lucrative to sell on the streets, prescription opiates actually represent a purer and potentially more addictive form of heroin.

This problem of heroin addiction stems directly from opiate prescriptions, and it is now affecting people of all races and socioeconomic backgrounds—a phenomenon that is vividly detailed in *Dreamland: The True Tale of America's Opiate Epidemic*, a 2015 award-winning book by journalist Sam Quinones.[57] Quinones shares the stories of real people whose lives fell from grace as they became unexpectedly addicted to opioid painkillers. When their prescriptions were threatened, many would "doctor shop," borrow pills from a friend, or buy them on the street or over the Internet. When these options ran out or became too expensive, many turned to the cheap, street alternative—heroin. When the musician Prince died from an accidental overdose in May 2016, his death drew considerable national attention to this epidemic.

Individuals who have been prescribed an opiate painkiller are forty times more likely to abuse or become dependent on heroin. In 2013, 169,000 Americans became first-time users of heroin. Between 2011 and 2013, heroin use in the United States increased among men and women, most age groups, and all income levels. In the same period, the number of heroin deaths doubled, claiming 120 deaths per day.[58]

In 2015, the CDC director summarized the problem this way:

> Heroin use is increasing at an alarming rate in many parts of society, driven by both the prescription opioid epidemic and cheaper, more available heroin. To reverse this trend we need an all-of-society response—to improve opioid prescribing practices to prevent addiction, expand access to effective treatment for those who are addicted, increase use of naloxone to reverse overdoses, and work with law enforcement partners like the DEA to reduce the supply of heroin.[59]

To be clear, opiates are essential to modern medicine. Many invasive and surgical procedures could not be performed without them, and they speed the recovery process by enabling patients to more quickly resume normal activities. Although powerful, these drugs can be safely used with most patients; however, getting the dosages properly titrated to a patient's medical and mental status could be improved with input from patients and family members—because even subtle changes in a patient's status can affect the safety of opiate drugs.

Unintended advanced sedation (overdosing) and respiratory distress from opiates can result in insufficient oxygen, pulmonary edema (swelling), hypothermia, and death.

Effectively managing opiate treatment in hospitals is challenging because how patients respond is influenced by a host of acute medical factors, including the length of time a patient spent under general anesthesia, the presence of other sedating drugs, any surgical incisions that may impair breathing, and the patient's general state of health. How opiates impact patients is also affected by preexisting conditions, such as sleep disorders, obesity, snoring, pulmonary and cardiac dysfunction or disease, smoking status, and age. Complicating things further, one of the vital signs used to titrate opiate doses is the patient's report of pain, which is an inherently subjective self-reported measure. A patient's history of substance abuse and addiction is another nonmedical factor that affects the safety of opiate treatment.

For a time, hospital use of the drug that brought Josie back from a state of serious oversedation—naloxone—was considered the "cost of doing business." Today, there is growing appreciation for the idea that the need for naloxone, in and of itself, constitutes a patient safety event. Like healthcare-associated infections, the need for hospitals to use naloxone can no longer be dismissed as a necessary ill.

Input from patients and patient advocates is centrally important to the safe use of opiates. To a degree, these drugs must be ordered based on the patient-reported felt need for the medications. Because patient input impacts how these drugs are used, they and their lay caregivers must be informed of the potential dangers of these medications, the signs of overdose and dependence, and what to do if they or their loved ones have concerns. With over half of all hospital patients receiving opiate drugs, there is a compelling reason to enlist patients and their lay caregivers in the process of accurately administering and monitoring them.

PAINKILLER PRECAUTIONS

When patients leave the hospital, there is far less ability to monitor patients' use of and response to these medications. Sending patients home from the hospital with unnecessary opiate prescriptions can create potentially serious problems for patients and/or those around them. The more an addictive drug is prescribed, the more likely it will be diverted and abused.[60]

Especially upon discharge, it is critical that patients and their lay caregivers understand the importance of using the least amount of opiate medication required, as well as the signs of opiate overdose and dependence, the dangers of mixing opiates with alcohol and other medications, and the fact that a personal and family history of alcohol and drug abuse may increase a person's chance of opiate abuse or diversion of their medications for misuse by themselves or others who have access to them. Simply asking patients if they have a history of alcohol or substance abuse is not a sufficient preventive measure.

Without adequate knowledge about why this question is asked, many patients fail to appreciate the importance of full disclosure.

A NURSE'S NIGHTMARE, ANYONE'S NIGHTMARE

Worldwide, up to thirty-six million people abuse prescription opiates, including about 1.5 million Americans over the age of twelve.[61] The problem has hit healthcare providers hard, especially nurses. *The Nurses* is an in-depth investigation of the working lives of hospital nurses and their shocking behind-the-scenes secrets by best-selling author Alexandra Robbins. The book follows a nurse who struggles with her addiction to opiates and history of taking doses prescribed for her patients. The author describes the tactics that nurses use to steal these medications from hospitals, nursing homes, hospice care centers, and other workplaces.[62] For example, nurses are supposed to "waste" (safely discard) patients' leftover pain medications, but it is easy for them to take them home. One nurse admitted to peeling pain patches off nursing home patients.[63] It is also easy for nurses to give patients only a portion of what is prescribed for them and pocket or shoot up the rest. Furthermore, a number of studies suggest that the problem is actually many times higher among nurses than the general population due to their chronic work-related stress and easy access to these powerful drugs. Robbins notes that the American Nurses Association estimates that 6 percent to 8 percent of nurses are now impaired at work due to substance abuse, often involving opiates.

The Nurses also includes this riveting side note: Jan Stewart, a twenty-eight-year certified nurse anesthetist who was president of the American Association of Nurse Anesthetists and widely respected and beloved by colleagues, suffered from addiction to opiates and died at the age of fifty from an opiate overdose. Nurse Stewart's addiction began with the painkillers she was prescribed after back surgery. Just as a main character in *The Goldfinch*,[64] a 2013 Pulitzer Prize–winning novel, nurses (and others) can appear to be functioning relatively normally while seriously abusing opiate drugs. Such may be true of other groups of employees, especially those whose jobs place them at high risk of being physically hurt or injured.

According to anonymous surveys colleagues and I collected in October 2016 from industrial workers from over fifty companies in Virginia, over 10 percent reported they sometimes take prescription pain medication to perform their jobs. While some percentage of the respondents may have been referring to the use of non-narcotic prescription pain medications, this is unlikely to be the case for the majority of them. A recent twenty-one-state analysis of treatment for work-related injuries that did not require surgery indicated that 78 percent of employees received opioids, with state rates ranging from a low of 60 percent (Connecticut) to a high of 90 percent (Arkansas). Although respondents to our Safety & Leadership Survey were not from one of the highest opioid use states, they were from the southeastern region of Virginia known as Hampton Roads, which has a documented problem with the overuse of opioids.[65] Moreover, the rate of opioid use among injured workers is high (60 percent or greater) even in states with comparatively low rates of opioid use.

The problem of opiate-heroin abuse can strike anyone, anywhere. Carolyn Weems was right to be worried about others suffering the same tragedy that her family must now endure. Between 1995 and 2002, the number of American teenagers who had used heroin increased 300 percent. So in 2015, Weems posted about the problem on the Virginia Beach City Public Schools website, wrote about it in the local newspaper, and convened a meeting of over two hundred parents and professionals from Virginia Beach to candidly discuss the issue.

In her crusade, Weems grabbed the attention of Virginia's attorney general, Mark Herring. Ever since, Weems and Herring have been dedicated to making the public aware that people of all ages, stages, and classes are using heroin. In 2014, more teens in Virginia died from heroin than from car accidents.[66] A 2015 investigation revealed that nine hundred nurses in Virginia were publicly disciplined for stealing drugs at work in the past few years.[67] The problem of opiate/heroin addiction is not limited to Virginia; it is a serious national epidemic. In fact, looking at the rate of opiate prescriptions by state, Virginia falls in the bottom half.[68]

We can, and must, do a better job of managing patient pain while averting such unacceptably high rates of opiate prescriptions, diversion, abuse, addiction, and death. Indeed, providers must familiarize themselves with the CDC opiate guidelines that were released in 2016 that promote judicious use of opioid painkillers;[69] however, solving the opioid/heroin epidemic will require a societal—not just medical—response. Moving forward, efforts to curb this epidemic will require dedication inside hospitals as well as in our communities.

In addition to providing a summary of key information (table 5.3), a patient action plan (table 5.4), and a sticky message with sample language for promoting safe medication administration (table 5.5), this chapter also offers a summary of key information about the safe management of opiate drugs (table 5.6).

Table 5.3.

WHAT YOU NEED TO KNOW
Medication Administration Errors

Information for Patients
Medication errors are common. Every patient is at high risk. On average, hospital patients experience one medical error per day. Such errors are even more common in nursing homes. Most hospitals use electronic health records and other technologies to reduce the chance of drug errors, but technology cannot catch all errors. Making sure you receive the correct drugs (and only those drugs) requires focused attention.

Whenever you are able to participate, nurses should invite you to verify your identity and review these Five Rights:

1	2	3	4	5
Right Patient	Right Drug	Right Dose	Right Route	Right Time

Information for Providers
Approximately 17 million drug errors occur in US hospitals each year. The rate of error is even higher in US nursing homes. Hospitals use various technologies to prevent drug errors, but technology is not perfect. It is only as good as the systems that support it and the people who use it. So, never allow yourself to develop a false sense of security because technology usually gets things right.

While there is no magic bullet for preventing all medication errors, two safety habits can eliminate many of them. Whenever possible involve patients to: (1) verify their identity and (2) review the Five Rights of Medication Administration. Doing so creates a two-person check without needing to track down another provider, and it has the potential to catch up to 95 percent of medication administration errors. |

Table 5.4.

PATIENT ACTION PLAN Medication Administration Errors		
TIMING	**PATIENT ACTION**	✓
ASAP	I created a written list of all my medications, including: ☐ prescription drug dosages, routes of delivery (oral, patch, etc.), and timing (how often I take it) ☐ over-the-counter drugs I take on a regular basis ☐ my name and date of birth	
	I am prepared to bring my medication list to all medical appointments and facilities where I will be treated.	
	I reviewed my medication list with a family member or friend and/or let someone know where I keep it, so they can help in an emergency.	
Before being admitted to a hospital	I know the Five Rights refer to the right: (1) patient, (2) drug, (3) dosage, (4) route, and (5) time.	
	I practiced what to say if a nurse or someone else attempts to give me a drug without reviewing the Five Rights with me.	
	I will expect my identity to be verified by two pieces of information before a drug is given—even if this must happen many times each day.	
	I will speak up whenever care providers: fail to introduce themselves, verify my ID, review the Five Rights with me; or if something doesn't seem right.	

Table 5.5.

WHAT YOU CAN SAY	
Sticky Message: **Safety Starts with a Name**	
When Someone Walks into a Patient Room without Introducing Himself or Herself	
Patient Request—Examples	**Desired Response—Examples**
"I'm glad you're here to help, but would you mind introducing yourself?"	"Forgive me for not introducing myself. My name is ___. I am a ___. I am here to ___."
"I know you're my nurse, but I've forgotten your name and I'm wondering what you're doing to my IV bag."	"My name is Laura. I will be your nurse until 10 p.m. and I am here to check your medications at the start of my shift. Sorry I didn't explain that when I walked in. How are you doing?"
Sticky Message: **ID Me Before You Treat Me**	
When Someone Wants to Do Something to You without Verifying Your ID	
Patient Request—Examples	**Desired Response—Examples**
"Nurse Mary, I know we're familiar with each other, but let's double-check my ID and review the order before you push drugs through my IV."	"Thank you, Mrs. Jones. This is a busy place. I don't want to let a mistake slip through the cracks."
"Mr. Brown, I'm eager to get my X-ray, but would you verify the name on the order before you transport me?"	"Absolutely! Thanks for checking. I meant to do that. Let's do that right now."
Sticky Message: **No Review, No Drugs**	
If Someone Attempts to Administer a Medication Before Reviewing It with You	
Patient Request—Examples	**Desired Response—Examples**
"It might have been reviewed before, but let's make sure we have the right patient and medication."	"Thank you for checking. Let's check that your wristband matches the order and review the order together. Let me know if anything is incorrect, if you have questions or something doesn't seem right about the drug, dose, method of delivery, or timing."
"Nurse Kevin, before you connect that medication bag, would you mind reviewing the order with me?"	"Of course! I love caring for patients who help make sure we get things right."
"Dr. Jones, as far as I know, there have been no changes to my medication, but let's review everything to make sure no mix-ups have occurred."	"Yes, let's do that right now. I am glad you're paying close attention to the medications you are getting."

Table 5.6.

WHAT YOU NEED TO KNOW
Opioid Painkillers

Information for Patients

Opioid painkillers are one of the most commonly prescribed medications. They are important for helping patients manage their pain, especially after surgeries and invasive procedures. Opiates can speed the recovery process by helping patients resume normal activities as soon as possible. However, these drugs are powerful, addictive, and overprescribed.

The need for painkillers is subjective, and the ability of patients to tolerate such drugs varies widely. Disclose any history of alcohol or drug abuse to your providers because this can affect your reaction to the medication. Always take as little pain medication as necessary. Although hospital providers do everything they can to monitor patient reactions to pain medications, patients are unique and patient status can change rapidly. Therefore, family and friends involved with your care must feel free to call attention to any signs that you may be overly sedated or dehydrated.

Even highly competent doctors and nurses can overlook important signs and symptoms. To the best of your ability, speak up if you feel unnecessarily sleepy, unresponsiveness, or dehydrated. Ask about nondrug treatments for pain and non-narcotic (nonopioid) pain medications. They can be as (or more) effective than opioids for treating chronic pain.

Information for Providers

Beginning in the 1990s, pharmaceutical companies and pain management experts promoted opioid painkillers as relatively nonaddictive, but we now recognize that opioid painkillers are highly addictive. They should be used sparingly and not as a first-line treatment for chronic pain.

Because opioid use has increased dramatically over the last five to ten years, opioid addiction now affects 2.5 million Americans on a daily basis. Once addicted, many people turn to inexpensive heroin when they cannot afford to obtain prescription opioids. In fact, 80 percent of heroin users first used opioids for pain relief.

In 2016, the CDC released a new opioid guideline. Familiarize yourself with its twelve specific recommendations to help you determine (a) when to initiate or continue opioids; (b) how to select, dosage, monitor, and discontinue opioids; and (c) how to assess opioid risks and harms.

CHAPTER 6

Beyond the Bedside

Improve Patient Safety One Community at a Time

A Deadly Chemotherapy Mix-Up

The mother said, "That doesn't look like the chemo she has gotten previously. Are you sure it's right?" She asked again a bit later. And she asked a third time. She was right and her child—who had a curable cancer—died of a chemotherapy mixture error. The nurse confirmed each time that the label on the bag was accurate. And each time, the nurse assured the mother it was the right medication. And she was right—the label said the right thing. But that wasn't what was in the bag.

I was responsible for the pharmacy and pharmacists who were the source of the error and resulting death of a lovely seven-year-old girl and the devastation of a mother who felt she didn't do enough to protect her child. As an organization, we were long in our safety journey and this horrific death showed us how far we had to go. Together with the pharmacy department team members, we faced the reality of what we had done and created a short list of terrible things never to be repeated.

—Roundtable participant, NPSF Lucien Leape Institute[1]

UNITED IN SAFETY

Every time I read the above excerpt, I cringe. This tragic chemotherapy mix-up exemplifies how easy it is for mistakes to occur and reminds us that patient concerns are too likely to be overlooked, even when they signal that a major patient safety event may be about to occur. Like the examples in previous chapters, this story exposes how devastating it can be for patients when basic human error slips through the cracks. It also reminds us that providers don't walk away unscathed.

With a vision to create a world where both "patients and those who care for them are free from harm," the National Patient Safety Foundation recently updated its strategic plan with four major goals. It now seeks to:

- Engage with Patients, Families, and Communities
- Engage the Healthcare Community
- Partner with Key Stakeholders
- Impact Healthcare Leaders and Policymakers

Furthermore, as of 2016, the foundation's theme became "United in Safety," meaning "*everyone* involved in the healthcare process plays a role in the delivery of safe care."[2]

This chapter introduces a well-established public health strategy that is tailor-made for operationalizing the foundation's vision. Although community coalitions have been largely ignored by the patient safety movement, they have a proven track record for addressing public health problems with characteristics just like patient safety's most pressing issues, which is why it is my hope that creating community-based patient safety coalitions and connecting their efforts with hospital-based initiatives becomes the next wave of the patient safety movement.

This chapter explains how community coalitions specific to patient safety can overcome existing barriers and why doing so represents an urgently needed strategy to kick-start a new wave of the movement.

THE ROAD TO HARM IS PAVED WITH GOOD INTENTIONS

What has been the fallout of healthcare's repeated failure to create patient advisories and engagement interventions that offer sufficient input from their target audience? According to an analysis conducted by a now former fellow at the Harvard School of Public Health, existing advisories—even those created by leading US healthcare organizations—generate unrealistic expectations.[3] Among other problems, they may create unreasonable demands on lay caregivers given people's schedules, preferences, and capabilities. Worse yet, some might precipitate a loss of confidence and trust in hospital care.[4] Consider the following information that has been extracted from prominent patient safety advisories.

Unrealistic Expectations—Example A

Ask a trusted family member or friend to stay with you, even overnight, when you are hospitalized. You will be able to rest more comfortably and your advocate can help to make sure you get the right medications and treatments. . . . If you do not recognize a medication, verify that it is for you. Ask about oral medication before swallowing, and read the bags of intravenous (IV) fluids. If you're not well enough to do this, ask your advocate to do this.[5]

Unrealistic Expectations—Example B

If you're going into the hospital . . . your most important step is selecting someone you trust to be your healthcare advocate. . . . The most important attribute for your healthcare advocate is the willingness and ability to speak up—to ask questions when things happen that you don't understand and to insist that people take the necessary measures to protect you from harm.[6]

It is easy to imagine how anxious a patient and/or family members might feel upon reading such information while in the hospital or shortly before someone is admitted. Raising public awareness about safety is important, but current approaches have done little to help people protect themselves or their loved ones. The availability of informational pamphlets certainly hasn't put a dent in the magnitude of the crisis.

What's more, the Harvard analysis also suggests that existing advisories may do more harm than good by exacerbating a lingering sense of guilt among patients and family members. When mishaps do occur, patients might be left feeling like they should have done more especially if they didn't speak up or believe they should have persisted longer when providers rebuffed their concerns. The advisories could also cause providers to view outspoken patients as "difficult patients" and allow this perception to influence the quality of their care.

Undoubtedly, patients can play a critical role in decreasing the occurrence of patient safety events—but the utmost care must be taken to prevent the perception that the healthcare industry wishes to *transfer* the burden of responsibility for safety to patients. Yes, hospitals and other healthcare organizations have an obligation to *invite* patients to engage in the process—for everyone's well-being—but healthcare organizations cannot demand that all patients become effective partners in safe care, nor can they blame patients when they fail to come to the aid of their providers.

I will never forget when a neurology colleague lambasted me for what he perceived as my causing patients to challenge his authority. This otherwise measured and kindly pediatrician stormed into my office one day and screamed, "You're causing patients to question my diagnosis. This needs to stop!" He also asked administrators of the medical school where we worked to cease and desist all media attention for my work that exposed the overuse of psychiatric drugs and threatened my career mobility. Although this occurred more than ten years ago, the experience is a potent reminder that unintended and negative consequences might befall patients and others who speak up for safety *unless* their providers are also prepared to view such actions in a positive light.

The health and functional ability of providers are also riding on the development of realistic patient-engagement strategies. Think about the various examples of tragic errors in this book. How can we meaningfully engage patients in safety initiatives without inappropriately shifting the burden of responsibility to them, without disrupting the patient-provider relationship, and without otherwise causing more harm than good?

LESSONS LEARNED FROM SOLVING OTHER TOUGH PROBLEMS

Insights about how to best engage patients and families (as well as providers) may be gleaned from the work of Jerry and Monique Sternin. As a couple, the Sternins spent their careers tackling complex public health problems around the world. In every instance, they discovered effective solutions by connecting with the people who were dealing with the problem on a personal level. In fact, this insight represents the prevailing message conveyed in the book that they coauthored with Richard Pascale, a global business consultant and associate fellow at

Oxford University's business school. *The Power of Positive Deviance* provides vivid and compelling examples of the power of ordinary people to come up with ingenious, inexpensive, and sustainable solutions to complex problems.[7]

As explained in *The Power of Positive Deviance*, the Sternins discovered that stubborn crises, like reducing childhood malnutrition in Vietnam and curbing the practice of female genital mutilation in Egypt, are best viewed as *adaptive problems*. Adaptive problems refer to issues that are (a) embedded in complex social systems and (b) require social and behavioral change to yield transformative results. Solving adaptive problems always requires getting people to break old social and behavioral patterns and replace them with new ones. Getting a handle on the "technical stuff" (specific practices and tools) is important, but it was never sufficient to counteract longstanding, culturally embedded social norms that sustain adaptive problems. The hardest part of the Sternins' work always involved making sure technical know-how was incorporated into daily routines.

Lesson One

Solving seemingly insurmountable public health issues often has less to do with figuring out what needs to be done and more to do with figuring out how to get people to do what needs to be done.

Positive deviance refers to a people-driven and bottom-up approach to solving seemingly insurmountable problems. It accepts as a given that solutions will be dependent on discovering what can and will work by connecting directly with those whose behavior needs to change. Positive deviance succeeds by first identifying those rare individuals who have managed to overcome a problem that is endemic to their environment. The Sternins referred to such shining stars as *positive deviants* because their behaviors deviated from cultural expectations in ways that enabled them to succeed against the odds. In each case, they discovered that leveraging positively deviant practices was key to mitigating the public health crisis. Invariably, the positively deviant practices involved actions that could be attained by anyone in the community and did not need to be forced on a community by outside experts.

Lesson Two

Paying attention to the rare few community members who seem to succeed against the odds brings to light solutions that would otherwise remain "invisible in plain sight."

After the Vietnam War, a variety of factors seriously undermined the country's rice production. As a result, by 1990, about two-thirds of all Vietnamese children under the age of five suffered from malnutrition. International feeding programs that temporarily improved the situation also engendered a sense of passiveness among the program beneficiaries. As soon as the programs ended, the villages relapsed into hunger. The Vietnamese government wanted the Sternins to help it create a lasting solution to the country's widespread problem of childhood malnutrition.

The Sternins began their work in Vietnam by searching for a few children who were thriving. Once found, they observed these families until they saw the solutions that had been invisible in plain sight. For example, in the positive deviant families, parents made sure that the young children were fed more than three times per day. It turns out that the young children could not finish their allotted food ration in one sitting. However, by increasing the number of meals they were fed each day, the thriving children ended up consuming a greater number of calories because they ate their entire ration. Unbeknownst to others in the community, the positively deviant families also added other foods to their children's meals—foods that were freely available to everyone but universally disdained (greens, shrimp, and crabs).[8] The successful practices of positively deviant families were accessible to all community members. In fact, some of the positive deviants were among the poorest families in their communities. That's what made them a turnkey solution to the widespread problem of malnutrition.

Lesson Three

When a broad segment of the population is affected by a given health problem, workable solutions must involve straightforward and inexpensive actions.

The Sternins then recruited volunteers to help measure and monitor progress in spreading the positive deviants' solutions to malnutrition. Within less than six months, the positively deviant practices had been widely embraced and more than 40 percent of the children in the Vietnamese villages were well nourished. Another 20 percent had moved from severe to moderate malnutrition. Rather than lecturing families, the Sternins and the volunteers provided concrete ways for families to experience the results of simple behavioral changes. Working together with other villagers, the local volunteers made sure that families were involved in weighing their children and monitoring their weight gain. Parents could see for themselves those families that embraced the positively deviant practices—including supplementing their children's meals with foods that had been considered off limits—had children who gained weight and thrived.

Lesson Four

It is sometimes easier to get people to act their way into a new way of thinking than to think their way into a new way of acting.

About ten years ago, a handful of healthcare professionals began taking note of the power of positive deviance; a few had the courage to test its mettle in the hospital setting.

NECESSITY IS THE MOTHER OF INVENTION

Dr. Jon Lloyd was responsible for reducing the spread of MRSA in the Veteran's Administration Pittsburgh Healthcare System, and he had become exasperated by his failed attempts to solve this problem. During this time, he learned about the positive deviance process. Recognizing that entrenched healthcare traditions and cultural norms made it difficult for staff to call out infection-spreading behaviors, he jumped on the idea that the positive deviance process might help identify and address other barriers to effective infection prevention. When asked about his decision to pursue the people-driven positive deviance approach, Lloyd said:

The US healthcare industry has been too focused, for too long, on fixing errors, too preoccupied with making right what is wrong. Nurses and hospital staff have been bombarded with a litany of top-down, expert-driven directives to fix a broken system.[9]

From the start, Lloyd was acutely aware that hospitals don't have the time or resources to allow their staff to participate in time-intensive, bottom-up work that is a keystone of the positive deviance approach. So, he thoughtfully compressed the positive deviance time frame by engaging hospital staff through *lightly facilitated conversations* with frontline workers to discover *solutions*. These conversations replaced the slower-paced, positive deviant process that the Sternins had used in their fieldwork in developing countries. As indicated in the table below, every facilitated conversation addressed six questions that were key to engaging a community and uncovering positive deviance.

Table 6.1.

Using Facilitated Conversations to Identify Solutions, MRSA Case Example	
The Problem	How do you know if your patient has MRSA or carries the germ?
Personal Experience	In your own practice, what do you do to prevent spreading MRSA to other patients and staff?
Barriers	What prevents you from doing these things all the time?
Positive Deviance	Is there anyone who has a way of doing things that helps them overcome these barriers?
Stakeholders	What ideas do you have about others with whom we should meet?
Volunteers	What can we do now—any volunteers?

Source: Karim Saad, "Discovery and Action Dialogues: A Tool for Getting Started," in *Shared Care: Partners for Patients*, edited by BC Patient Safety & Quality Council, 2013.

To maximize involvement, Lloyd and his team invited the entire hospital staff to participate. They ended up facilitating conversations with five hundred staff members; each conversation lasted fifteen to twenty minutes. Through these conversations, staff quickly generated over one hundred ideas, including many viable solutions. Although they didn't originally plan to elicit patient input, Lloyd also invited patients from one of the hospital units to offer suggestions. This, too, resulted in valuable suggestions. For example, one patient suggested moving hand-sanitizing dispensers from the walls behind patient beds to the walls across from them so that patients could monitor whether staff washed their hands—a change that not a single staff member had considered, but one that proved to be extremely helpful.

In less than eighteen months, Lloyd and his colleagues identified and implemented a set of solutions that had been invisible in plain sight. As a result, the hospital reduced its overall MRSA infection rate by 50 percent (and by 70 percent in one particular unit). So, while national MRSA transmission rates were increasing fivefold, they were rapidly decreasing in Lloyd's hospital. If you recall the figures discussed previously, a 50 percent reduction in MRSA would translate to a financial savings of at least $2 million annually in direct cost-savings for an average-sized hospital[10] and the avoidance of a great deal of human suffering. Having observed how the process took hold and became self-sustaining, Lloyd said, "It's like letting the genie out of the bottle—you can't put it back in."[11]

Praise belongs to Dr. Lloyd for bravely adapting and testing such a novel approach in the hospital where he worked and for subsequently promoting its use in other hospitals. Five of the seventeen other hospitals in the VA Pittsburgh Healthcare System chose to apply to receive training in positive deviance, as did five VA hospitals in other states. The Department of Veteran Affairs and the Agency for Healthcare Research and Quality acknowledged the success of Lloyd's work, and the Institute for Healthcare Improvement continues to showcase it on its website.

Given the impressive reduction in the rate of MRSA that positive deviance work generated for the VA Pittsburgh Healthcare System, it is important to address what may be contributing to the seemingly slow and apparently limited diffusion of such innovation in other healthcare organizations. A recent literature search failed to reveal that the positive deviance approach has been practiced in US hospitals to the extent that one might expect, with little new information appearing since 2008.[12]

ACCELERATING PROGRESS

It is possible that the positive deviance practices that have worked so beautifully in developing countries are simply too out of sync with normal operations of most modern hospitals. In fact, it is a labor- and time-intensive approach that has had mixed success with large corporations.[13] The great news is that, in industrial countries like the United States, community coalitions have already proven to be an effective strategy for discovering and disseminating people-driven solutions, and they do so without disrupting hospital operations. For thirty years, they have been used to address a wide range of complex public health issues, such as teen smoking, childhood immunization rates, car seat safety, and the prevention of a variety of chronic health issues.[14]

A *community coalition* represents an alliance of local groups that share a common desire to make a positive change in their community. Community coalitions represent a blend of grassroots coalitions (which usually form around an acute crisis and last for a limited period of time) and professional coalitions or taskforces (which typically focus on state or national legislation and policy issues). Community coalitions bring together diverse groups and individuals to solve local problems.[15] Rather than addressing issues that may affect just one sector of the population, they focus on changes that benefit the entire community.[16] Without taking sole ownership for a broadly defined problem, community coalitions enable organizations to tackle issues through the use of pooled community knowledge and resources. The resulting synergy makes it possible to accomplish goals that no single organization could achieve on its own.[17] Community coalitions act as a catalyst for change among participating organizations and thereby influence the services provided to individuals, but they do not provide direct services themselves.

For more than five years, the US Agency for Healthcare Research and Quality and the nonprofit organization Consumers Advancing Patient Safety have advocated for the creation of local patient safety coalitions. To date, however, community-based patient safety coalitions remain conspicuously absent. Of note, some state and national patient safety organizations exist that have the word *coalition* in their names and/or mention consumers in their mission statements; however, these organizations are generally professional policy-oriented groups that function more like taskforces. They are distinctly different from community-based coalitions, which actively recruit members of the general public for full-level participation and emphasize two-way collaboration between those who deliver and receive care.

THE MISSING LINK

Think about the current reality. Technical requirements for reducing healthcare-associated infections, off-the-mark procedures, and medication administration errors are well known. These solutions involve consistent use of basic safety behaviors that are accessible to all healthcare workers. What has not yet been discovered is how to get providers to do what needs to be done. The key to making giant leaps forward, therefore, lies in discovering how to turn essential safety behaviors into consistent safety habits. It is these habits that represent healthcare's *keystone habits*—the small set of safety habits that can lead to transformative progress toward eliminating the most prevalent and predictable hospital safety events. As keystone habits, a few behavioral routines stand to have a disproportionate influence on progress relative to their cost and simplicity. Rather than getting millions of people to focus on a gazillion half-measures, traction around the keystone habits represents the sort of campaign that is needed.

Because the breadth and volume of healthcare providers who must consistently exhibit patient safety's keystone habits are so great—as are the breadth and volume of citizens who must help them get there—a people-driven, problem-solving strategy is imperative. In the United States, community coalitions excel at this kind of work. They are effective in raising public awareness and mobilizing coordinated efforts to engage the general public and healthcare providers around specific, desirable, and concrete actions.

A COALITION IN ACTION

The story of a coalition that succeeded may clarify how powerful they can be for mobilizing wide-scale change. Local patient safety coalitions are still rare; in fact, a recent and comprehensive review of the literature that was funded by the Agency for Healthcare Research and Quality identified only two articles that represented public health campaigns around patient safety. Given the lack of evidence to draw from, I offer a summary of my experience working with a school health coalition.

As a newly minted clinical psychologist, I joined a multidisciplinary team at the Naval Hospital in San Diego. The clinic rarely saw children who had been diagnosed with attention-deficit/hyperactivity disorder (ADHD), and our team rarely handed out that diagnosis. Four years later, when my family relocated to Virginia Beach, my Naval Hospital boss had retired from the military and was in the process of setting up a comparable clinic at the pediatric hospital located in the Norfolk-Virginia Beach area. He recruited me to join his practice, where I again participated in multidisciplinary team evaluations. But this time things were different. Seventy-five percent of the children we saw had been diagnosed with ADHD or were referred to rule out that diagnosis. It also seemed that everywhere I went, from my daughter's soccer practice to neighborhood cocktail parties, people were talking about ADHD. Believing that the condition was being terribly overdiagnosed by clinicians throughout the region (a region referred to as Hampton Roads and/or Coastal Virginia), I began asking questions and sharing my concerns with colleagues. Someone encouraged me to speak with one of the area public health directors, and she suggested that I form a coalition to address the problem.

With no prior coalition experience, I got together with others to form what came to be called the School Health Initiative for Education (SHINE). Throughout the time that SHINE existed, the question of whether children were being overmedicated for ADHD was a matter of intense national debate. Progress toward reducing overdiagnosis and treatment would have been impossible except that the coalition had engaged key stakeholders with diverse interests and perspectives. Consistent with the steps outlined in the table toward the end of this chapter,[18] SHINE members "got together" (Step 1) and asked me to serve as the coalition's chair. Next, SHINE members "got the real picture" (Step 2). They collected evidence that the community was undeniably an "ADHD hotspot."[19] Specifically, they gathered evidence that the rate of diagnosis and treatment had spun out of control, including documenting that Coastal Virginia cities were in the top 1 percent for national rates of ADHD drug treatment.[20] Rather than waiting for our research data to be published, SHINE "got connected" (Step 3) and became a vehicle for sharing the evidence of overdiagnosis throughout Coastal Virginia in a timely fashion.

With the help of a steering group, SHINE "got focused" (Step 4) by creating a mission statement and establishing its major goals. It "got organized" (Step 5) by establishing a regular schedule for workgroups and general meetings. These meetings were used to support, organize, and/or facilitate parent, teacher, and provider surveys, focus groups, key informant interviews, and analysis of new and extant databases. Based on the resulting community needs assessment, the coalition identified four major gaps in ADHD care: systematic behavior management in schools, school-provider communication, teacher training and education, and parent training and support. These were not the same issues that any one person or group would have independently identified as most important, nor were they topics that would have received widespread support had they not been generated with input from the community coalition: parents, teachers, clinical providers, school administrators, and other interested parties.

Everyone "got to work" (Step 6). With support and input from the community, my colleagues and I were able to write winning grant proposals and quickly secure local, state, and federal grant support to implement and evaluate the effectiveness of interventions for each of the community's self-identified gaps. SHINE's support from diverse community factions also made local officials more amenable to us conducting research and intervention projects in their school districts— something that often represents an insurmountable barrier to researchers. In addition to writing letters of support for funding applications, SHINE members served as an advisory group for research and intervention projects, monitoring progress and helping to remove barriers to their success when necessary.

One of our federally funded projects was a schoolwide, positive discipline program. It resulted in ADHD symptoms decreasing among elementary school students from the beginning to the end of the school year. This project also documented that teachers who adopted positive classroom management strategies had students who scored significantly higher in every subject area of the Standards of Learning tests administered to public school students across the state of Virginia.[21] SHINE members assisted with removing obstacles to piloting a program to facilitate communication (with parental permission) between parents and providers of children who were diagnosed with and/or treated for ADHD. The coalition also developed the single-page ADHD Diagnostic Checklist to remind or apprise parents, school personnel, and providers of the necessary steps to completing a comprehensive ADHD diagnostic assessment process—a handout that they prepared for distribution in clinics and schools throughout the region. They also created easy-to-read School Health Bulletins that were endorsed by the Virginia Department of Education and made available to parents and educators in schools around the region. And SHINE members successfully developed a bill that was passed by the Virginia Legislature that prohibited teachers from recommending ADHD medication to parents.

Finally, the SHINE coalition also "got proof" (Step 7) that their efforts had worked. From about 2000 to 2004, the Coastal Virginia region witnessed a 32 percent decrease in the rate of ADHD diagnosis and drug treatment—something that was not happening in other parts of the country.[22] While powerful pharmaceutical marketing campaigns were contributing to the overdiagnosis of ADHD nationally, the SHINE coalition was able to substantially reduce the number of children in Coastal Virginia who were diagnosed with the condition.[23] (Anyone who is familiar with mental health trends can appreciate how extraordinary it was that Coastal Virginia cut the number of children who were diagnosed with ADHD by one-third.)

Interestingly, parents in the Coastal Virginia region had reported greater satisfaction with behavioral interventions than drug treatment, although their children were far more likely to receive drug treatment than other interventions. To expand participation in parent training, local researchers and practitioners secured local, state, and federal funding to develop and implement a unique approach to marketing parenting classes. The program—the A+ Behavior Program: Helping Your Student Excel in School and at Home—experienced unprecedented levels of parent participation. It was so well received that all five districts in southeastern Virginia subsequently arranged for their psychologists and/or guidance counselors to receive training and supervision to deliver the program throughout the region. Some of the participants in this train-the-trainer program were affiliated with the Virginia Beach City Public Schools clinical psychology internship program and, together with SHINE members, created the first-ever public health psychology internship in the country—a program that was approved by the American Psychological Association.

That an innovative parenting program quickly morphed into a train-the-trainer initiative that was supported by five school districts with a goal of establishing a program in every elementary school across a region with a population of over 1.7 million and helped to spearhead the formation of the first-ever public health psychology internship program represents the sort of spontaneous accelerations of progress that coalitions and positive deviance efforts are known to generate. Without the SHINE coalition, barriers to appropriate care and solutions for reducing ADHD overdiagnosis and overtreatment that the community identified, supported, and evaluated might have remained invisible in plain sight. The coalition created opportunity for giant leaps forward in the delivery of evidence-based care to children with school-related behavioral problems.

While Coastal Virginia was reducing the rate of ADHD drug treatment among its children, the problem was escalating in other areas of the country. In 2013, the Centers for Disease Control and Prevention finally acknowledged that the debate about ADHD overdiagnosis had been settled; undeniably, ADHD was being overdiagnosed in communities in every single state.[24] One of the leading industry-funded professionals who had long advocated for expanding ADHD diagnosis and drug treatment—an author of one of the most popular ADHD diagnostic instruments—also finally spoke out. Clinical psychologist C. Keith Conners, professor emeritus at Duke University, declared ADHD drug treatment to be a "disastrous epidemic of dangerous proportions."[25] By then, so many misdiagnosed children had been growing up and showing up on college campuses with stimulant drugs in hand that the country was experiencing an epidemic of ADHD drug abuse and addiction among college students and young adults.[26] However, also by then, thanks to efforts of SHINE, Coastal Virginia communities were no longer leading the nation with respect to ADHD overdiagnosis and associated drug treatment. Had the coalition "gotten recognized" properly (Step 8), its successes may have spread to other communities. Reasons why this did not occur have been documented in "Shooting the Messenger: The Case of ADHD," an article that is freely available on the Internet.[27]

Table 6.2.

	PUBLIC ACTION PLAN	
	Build Local Patient Safety Coalitions	
1	**Get Together**	Convene a meeting of people interested in the topic of patient safety and use the opportunity to share ideas with other members of your community who might be able to help form and guide a coalition.
2	**Get a Real Picture**	Establish a steering group that represents your community's diverse interests in patient safety, making sure that the group is capable of gathering data to paint a realistic picture of the problem at the local level.
3	**Get Connected**	Brainstorm and leverage all available organizations and groups in your community that are interested in improving patient safety, have knowledge about improving safety or health outcomes, or have a strong sense of civic responsibility. Create a system to ensure that all interested parties are informed about the work of the coalition. Recruit a core group of citizen members.
4	**Get Focused**	Narrow in on the aspect(s) of patient safety that the coalition will address initially and develop a mission statement to give everyone a sense of what you are working toward.
5	**Get Organized**	Establish major coalition goals and related working groups. Collaboratively decide what strategies will logically reduce the identified problem(s), and how you will measure, monitor, and report progress.
6	**Get to Work**	Create an action plan that defines who does what, by when, and how. Recruit additional members and volunteers as needed.
7	**Get Proof**	Gather information to determine whether you produced the amount of change desired by the coalition. Assess what strategies worked well, which ones were not effective, and next steps.
8	**Get Recognized**	Share your success. Announce your achievements through the coalition and the media, soliciting new members to sustain and expand coalition efforts as appropriate.

TAKING STOCK AND MUSTERING COURAGE

Almost anybody with a passion to improve patient safety can serve as the impetus for making positive change in his or her community. When I initiated conversations about ADHD overdiagnosis in my community, I was shy, reserved, and terrified of public speaking. I knew nothing about conducting community needs assessments, how coalitions operated, or that such things even existed. At the start, it is not essential to have a detailed understanding of how coalitions operate or how to get them funded. Plenty of information and people are available to guide the process once this becomes a decided course of action.

For anyone who wants to champion the formation of a community coalition, it may be helpful to have a summary of what we've learned about the patient safety crisis from a public health perspective.

The Crisis

- Medical errors are now a leading cause of death in the United States.[28] Every hour, nearly forty patients in US hospitals die as a result of preventable healthcare-induced harm, resulting in billions of dollars of excess healthcare costs every year.
- Healthcare-associated infections, off-the-mark procedures, and medication administration errors represent three of the most prevalent, predictable, and preventable types of patient safety events.

Human Error

- Healthcare's most prevalent, predictable, and preventable patient safety events are tied to simple human errors.
- Every provider is prone to commit the sort of errors that contribute to the most prevalent, predictable, and preventable patient safety events.

Safety-Critical Habits

- Simple and essentially cost-free safety habits exist that have the potential to prevent the most prevalent, predictable, and preventable patient safety events.
- Environmental cues help everyone form and maintain safety habits, but the healthcare industry has a long history of downplaying the need for such prompts.
- Patients have the potential to cue providers about safety habit oversights at critical junctures during the care process, but they have not been adequately prepared to serve in this capacity.

- Providers have the capacity to respond positively when patients speak up when they observe specific safety oversights, but they have not been adequately prepared to do so.

Effective Patient-Provider Engagement

- Raising public awareness about the patient safety crisis is an important first step in engaging patients and their families; however, other supports must be in place to help patients and family members use the information to speak up for safety and to ensure providers respond effectively.
- Public health strategies are most powerful when they are tailored to meet the social, cultural, and economic reality, priority, and capacity of a given community.

Community-Based Patient Safety Coalitions

- Community-based coalitions are a proven method for raising public awareness and pooling resources to identify, implement, and evaluate community-responsive solutions to public health problems.
- Nonprofit and government agencies have advocated for the formation of community-based patient safety coalitions, but they remain conspicuously absent.

Essential Pieces of the Puzzle

- Medical research has identified critical safety habits that, if used consistently, can drastically reduce or eliminate the trifecta of issues that comprise patient safety's low-hanging fruit—healthcare-associated infections, off-the-mark procedures, and medication administration errors.
- Behavioral science (psychology) has taught us what needs to be done to establish desirable habits and to make them stick.
- Public health has established that community-based coalitions and related strategies are effective for mobilizing and coordinating changes in patient and provider behaviors.

It is tempting to detail how a community might tackle the crisis, but communities vary greatly in terms of capacity and resources to support a coalition, so it is not wise to do so. Moreover, greater joy, ingenuity, and sustainability are likely to ensue when communities decide for themselves which issues they want to tackle and then determine what will work for their particular circumstances. There is no right answer, but there is a universally urgent need to uncover solutions that are currently invisible in plain sight.

TAKING ACTION

Sometimes community coalitions form at the local level and are then replicated across broader geographic regions with financial support being secured through a hodge-podge of mechanisms. In other instances, a national organization serves as the instrument for forming local coalitions by providing funding to communities throughout the country, as happened, for example, with a portion of the funding from the 1998 Tobacco Master Settlement Agreement.

From the very beginning, the National Patient Safety Foundation has been a central voice in the patient safety movement, and its current direction is consistent with the idea of creating community coalitions to accelerate progress. More than any other agency or organization, this foundation may be ideally positioned to facilitate and support the formation of community coalitions in communities around the United States. Furthermore, in 2007, the National Patient Safety Foundation formed an institute for a purpose that supports the ideas expressed in this book:

> The NPSF Lucien Leape Institute was formed in 2007 to provide strategic vision for improving patient safety. Composed of national thought leaders with a common interest in patient safety, the Institute functions as a think tank to identify new approaches to improving patient safety, call for the innovation necessary to expedite the work, create significant, sustainable improvements in culture, process, and outcomes, and encourage key stakeholders to assume significant roles in advancing patient safety.[29]

As a think tank, the Lucien Leape Institute could serve as the repository of lessons learned and thereby the vehicle to expedite the diffusion of innovation. Equally important, the institute could become the one-stop resource for technical support to help communities understand how to build effective patient safety coalitions. Many other nonprofit organizations could be equally appropriate national champions or sponsors, perhaps especially Leapfrog or the National Business Coalition on Health, because they too are heavily invested in the consumer side of improving patient safety.

BABY STEPS AND GIANT LEAPS

By the time you read this book, perhaps a national organization will have come onboard with the idea of supporting the formation of patient safety coalitions in communities across the United States. Regardless, there is no reason to wait. All it takes to get started is to have a conversation with others to discover who else might be able to help champion patient safety improvements in your own backyard. You may discover people who have prior coalition experience or other relevant experience. Although it is overused, there is a famous Margaret Meade quote that sums up the message of this chapter:

> Never doubt that a small group of thoughtful committed citizens can change the world; indeed, it's the only thing that ever has.

Admittedly, the idea of bringing members of competing healthcare facilities together with patients and other members of the public may be threatening to business and community leaders. Healthcare is a competitive business, and there are a variety of metrics over which healthcare organizations in any given community must and will compete, including certain safety metrics. Recall that, as discussed in the beginning of this book, The Leapfrog Group pushes for greater transparency around hospital safety metrics as a way to allow market forces to trigger giant leaps forward in the journey toward safe care.

Although competition is healthy and can spur innovation, there are also circumstances and issues over which cooperation—rather than competition—is in the best interests of everyone. Selecting a single patient safety issue to bring key stakeholders together is likely to increase their willingness to cooperatively seek solutions that affect everyone in the community. One of the few community-oriented efforts to improve patient safety was organized by Dr. Kathleen Leonhardt of Aurora Health Care.[30] Leonhardt indicated that selecting a single issue created a turning point in collaboration among otherwise competitive organizations.[31]

When a community discovers workable solutions to one of its seemingly insurmountable patient safety problems, it will have strengthened its capacity and resolve to tackle other issues in due time—provided that the unique interests of each member organization were respected along the way. Meanwhile, the building of local patient safety coalitions may be the best—or perhaps the only—way to more rapidly create a community where patients and those who care for them are free from harm.

Building community coalitions to facilitate the adoption of a more patient-centric view of safety and to identify workable solutions may seem like a tall order, but the rewards for doing so would be great. Consider how Dr. James L. Reinertsen, a prominent healthcare consultant and former CEO of Beth Israel Deaconess Medical Center in Boston, summarized the value of genuine patient engagement:

> We have observed that in a growing number of instances where truly stunning levels of improvement have been achieved, organizations have asked patients and families to be directly involved in the process. And those organizations' leaders often cite this change—putting patients in a position of real power and influence, using their wisdom and experience to redesign and improve care systems—as being the single most powerful transformational change in their history. Clearly, this is a leverage point where a small change can make a huge difference.[32]

Ironically, much of the work necessary to improve patient safety within hospitals and other healthcare facilities must occur outside these organizations through public health initiatives. Local patient safety coalitions fit the bill. They can raise awareness, motivate civic action, and offer hospital patients manageable steps to ensure safer care for themselves and others. The best return on investment may be realized by first addressing the most prevalent, predictable, and preventable types of patient safety events. Doing so will require a paradigm shift that will unify efforts from healthcare systems, public health, and society overall.

If you've read this far, you care about patient safety. Hopefully, you will initiate a conversation about the need to improve patient safety with at least one other person who lives or works in your community. If the two of you continue to have conversations about this pressing public health crisis until one or both of you encounters someone who—by virtue of position, knowledge, resources, or connections—can help create a patient safety coalition in your community, you will have taken small steps that can clear the path for giant leaps toward creating a world where patients and those who care for them are free from harm.

In the words of the National Patient Safety Foundation: "We need to mobilize. We are all in this together. Let's get the work done now."[33]

CHAPTER 7

Acceptance, Apology, and Forgiveness

Safeguard the Lives of Patients and Healthcare Providers

It is a capital mistake to theorize before one has data.

—Arthur Conan Doyle, *Memoirs of Sherlock Holmes*[1]

There could be no progress until enough people could be made dissatisfied—and this could be done only when they were brought to think beyond the limits to which they were accustomed.

—Thomas Edison, American inventor (1847–1931)[2]

Nurse Hiatt

Kimberly Hiatt had twenty-four years of nursing experience, impressive credentials, and numerous certifications when her employing hospital praised her as a "leading performer." Two weeks later, Kimberly mistakenly administered 1.4 grams of calcium chloride ($CaCl_2$) to an eight-month-old infant. That dose was ten times greater than what was ordered. Kimberly's mistake stemmed from a calculation error she made while being distracted by conversation with a coworker, which led her to confuse 1.4 grams and 140 milligrams. As soon as Kimberly discovered the error, she reported it to the staff and documented it in the hospital's electronic record system: "I messed up. I've been giving CaCl for years. I was talking to someone while drawing it up. Miscalculated in my head the correct mls according to the mg/ml. First med error in 25 yrs. of working here. I am simply sick about it. Will be more careful in the future." Several days after this event, the baby died. Although it was not clear that Kimberly's error caused the baby's death, the hospital fired her. When the state's nursing board learned of Kimberly's error, they required her to pay a fine to the board and placed her on a four-year probationary period, during which time she was required to be supervised while dispensing medication. Not surprisingly, Kimberly had difficulty finding another job. A few months after being fired and unable to secure a new position, Kimberly committed suicide.[3]

THE RIPPLE EFFECT

Initially there were only going to be six chapters in this book, but the more I talked about how common human error is in healthcare, the more necessary it was to foster appreciation for how devastating mistakes can be for healthcare providers, how often adverse outcomes stem from honest error, and how misguided it is to rush to judgment about who or what was responsible for the harm that sometimes befalls patients. *Your Patient Safety Survival Guide* is about uniting patients and healthcare providers to safeguard lives—not about inducing a sense of helplessness or misplaced anger. It would have been incomplete without this final chapter about inviting patients and providers to consider constructive actions they can take when patient safety events occur.

If you Google the Nurse Hiatt case, you will come across a photograph of Kimberly in her nursing scrubs; looking vibrant, fit, and happy—the very sort of image that might come to mind when you think about a competent nurse and a "leading performer." The photo does not depict a person you would expect to be fired or to commit suicide; however, in the absence of support, a patient safety event can have tragic consequences for any provider. Recent analyses indicate that following an adverse event, the majority of providers experience psychological distress, some seriously contemplate leaving the field, and a small portion never recover.[4] This ripple effect, called the *second victim phenomenon*, refers to a period of intense or prolonged anguish or guilt that results from witnessing or contributing to an event that caused harm to a patient.[5]

It was a Johns Hopkins physician—Albert Wu, MD—who first introduced the medical field to the second victim phenomenon. Later (in the same year that *To Err Is Human* was published), Wu courageously broke the longstanding silence about the agony providers feel in the face of a medical error, giving voice to their previously concealed vulnerability.

Provider Agony in the Face of Error

Virtually every practitioner knows the sickening realization of making a bad mistake. You feel singled out and exposed—seized by the instinct to see if anyone has noticed. You agonize about what to do, whether to tell anyone, what to say. Later, the event replays itself over and over in your mind. You question your competence but fear being discovered. You know you should confess, but dread the prospect of potential punishment and of the patient's anger. You may become overly attentive to the patient or family, lamenting the failure to do so earlier and, if you haven't told them, wondering if they know.

Sadly, the kind of unconditional sympathy and support that are really needed are rarely forthcoming. While there is a norm of not criticizing, reassurance from colleagues is often grudging or qualified. . . .

Further, there are no institutional mechanisms to aid the grieving process. Even when mistakes are discussed at morbidity and mortality conferences, it is to examine the medical facts rather than the feelings of the patient or physician. In the absence of mechanisms for healing, physicians find dysfunctional ways to protect themselves. They often respond to their own mistakes with anger and projection of blame, and may act defensively or callously and blame or scold the patient or other members of the healthcare team. . . . My observation is that this number includes some of our most reflective and sensitive colleagues, perhaps most susceptible to injury from their own mistakes.[6]

Later, a director of the Agency for Healthcare Research and Quality reinforced the importance of attending to the second victim phenomenon, describing it as a wounding burden:

The burden that healthcare providers feel after a patient is harmed, manifesting in anxiety, depression, and shame, weighs so heavily on providers that they themselves are wounded by the event.[7]

Because involvement in patient safety events harms the people who are available to care for us in our hours of need and because such involvement can negatively impact their ability to care for subsequent patients, some have described caring for second victims to be a moral imperative.[8] Engendering a sense of duty to care for providers whose actions contribute to serious patient safety events requires that we relinquish the unrealistic notion that our healthcare providers and the systems in which they work allow them to consistently perform without error.

LETTING GO OF UNREALISTIC EXPECTATIONS

It is important to remember that every human being makes mistakes. That means every healthcare provider will make mistakes. Anyone who cares for enough patients will eventually be involved in a seriously harmful mistake. In fact, a recent national survey of hospital-based pediatricians and pediatric residents found that 93 percent of them acknowledged having been personally involved in an error at some point during their training or career.[9] Think about it: if a hospital provider were to see an average of four patients in a twelve-hour shift (a low caseload), in a twenty-year career he or she will have cared for over eleven thousand patients.[10] This means that virtually every hospital provider will be involved in numerous patient safety events, some of which will have devastating consequences. In fact, 40 percent of today's providers report that they have been involved in a patient safety event in the past year, and some evidence suggests the rate may be even higher.[11]

Just because human error is inevitable and will, at times, cause serious harm to patients, healthcare has not let itself off the hook. To the contrary, as discussed in chapters 1 and 2, for the past two decades the industry has been diligently seeking to eliminate harm stemming from common human error. By the same token, just because it is theoretically possible to build safeguards into a system to catch errors, every medical error doesn't necessarily represent negligence on the part of the system or its providers. In a timeless paper, medical ethicist Samuel Gorovitz and world-renowned moral philosopher Alasdair MacIntyre reasoned why a just and fair response to healthcare-induced harm must be evaluated against the state of scientific knowledge.[12] In essence, Gorovitz and MacIntyre argue that as the state of scientific or medical knowledge improves over time, so too must our view of what constitutes negligence evolve.

Healthcare-associated infections are a clear case in point. Today, each infection that a patient picks up during the course of their hospital care is considered to be a patient safety event. Yet for more than one hundred years after we knew how to prevent the spread of most of these infections, the industry wrote them off as the cost of doing business. As a psychologist and public health practitioner, I have always been interested in how scientific knowledge is translated into routine clinical practice. This turns out to be a slow, uneven, and imperfect process. Just because a researcher has published a study that demonstrates how to eliminate a certain type of patient harm doesn't mean that every professional will immediately have a working knowledge of that discovery—a point that is driven home by the fact that Americans receive evidence-based care barely more than half the time.[13]

In today's world, translating medical discoveries into medical practice is complicated by the volume and complexity of the scientific literature. As of 2012, there were approximately twenty-eight thousand scholarly journals that publish close to two million scientific, technical, and medical articles per year—about half of which are in English.[14] To further understand this complexity, Professor MacIntyre recently reminded me of the incredibly important and relevant work by the world's premier scientists. Among other things, John P. A. Ioannidis is famous for demonstrating the troubling fact that half of all medical research claims that get published can be proven to be false.[15] Consider also that relatively few physicians read original scientific papers or have been adequately prepared to critique published results. This reality is conveyed in two compelling books about modern medicine: *Overtreated* by Shannon Brownlee and *Doctored* by Sandeep Jauhar.[16] So perhaps it should not be hard to comprehend why patients receive evidence-based care only about half the time they seek treatment. Over forty years ago, Gorovitz and MacIntyre said that we need a "more rational societal response to the reality of errors in clinical practice"[17] and this is all the more true today (arguably we also need a better way to ensure that clinical providers become more proficient at applying true medical and scientific discoveries).[18]

Here is a bit of medical history to put into perspective how scientific knowledge becomes common practice. In 1961, 90 percent of physicians surveyed preferred not to tell cancer patients about their diagnosis; by

1977, 97 percent felt the opposite. The shift from shielding patients from knowing their diagnosis to teaching them about it had virtually nothing to do with research or policy. The shift was facilitated principally by a change in physician training.[19] This shift reinforces the observation that determining culpability requires a great deal more consideration than the state of scientific knowledge.

We must also consider whether the behavior in question deviated from the accepted performance standard for the person's profession and/or employer. This requires that we ask a host of questions: Did the individuals involved in a patient safety event have (or should they have had) sufficient exposure to the ideal practice standard vis-à-vis their professional education, on-the-job training, or continuing education courses? Did the facility where the error occurred have (or should it have had) relevant policy or practice standards in place? Were there mitigating factors that prevented the individual from behaving in a manner that was consistent with the ideal standards and/or hospital policy? Or, more basic: Would most anyone have done the same thing under the same circumstances?

Returning to Kimberly Hiatt, here is what a retired physician wrote about the incident in *The Seattle Times*.

Managing Error in Medicine

One of the well-accepted principles of error management in medicine today is that mistakes are most commonly the result of system problems, not mere negligence on the part of the provider . . . If we fire everybody in medicine who makes an error, we will soon have no providers. We all make errors. It is only by the grace of God that most of them do not result in great harm or death. It is my belief that if the nurse had been dealt with appropriately—with compassion and insight—that she, today, would be a valuable and happy nurse. But she was fired. I, in no way, want to minimize the tragedy of the death of this infant, however, the death of Kimberly Hiatt is no less tragic.[20]

The physician's public commentary nailed it. We all make errors. Our errors rarely result from the willful disregard for others. Factors beyond the control of providers often influence the emergence of error, and, when errors occur, providers are often in need of compassion—

just like the event's primary victims. If we continue to place healthcare providers on pedestals of infallibility, they are guaranteed to fall from grace and leave us feeling excessively disappointed.

THE LURE OF HINDSIGHT

Not only do healthcare providers typically not receive compassion after being involved in a patient safety event, their employers, peers, and patients often avoid or reject them. While it may be reasonable to expect an overtly angry response from patients and families (especially after the immediate shock begins to wear off), colleagues and institutions can and must display greater equipoise and compassion. Even when a provider's action (or lack of action) appears to be in the wrong, our initial impression of what went wrong is apt to fall prey to the subtle but insidious problem of hindsight bias.

Hindsight bias refers to the knew-it-all-along phenomenon in which an event seems obvious when looking back with more facts in hand, although somewhat unpredictable with what was known at the time of the incident. In their groundbreaking book *Wall of Silence*, Rosemary Gibson and Janardan Prasad Singh recounted a sad but true story of three nurses who were wrongfully convicted in the minds of others before considering all the relevant facts.

The Denver Case

In a Denver hospital, a newborn infant died as a result of a medication error. Three nurses who were taking care of the infant were indicted for criminally negligent homicide. Two of the nurses accepted a guilty plea, the terms of which included a two-year probationary period, because they didn't want the third nurse, who had a negligible role in the error, to be found guilty by association. Experts on medical errors who were helping the nurse who stood trial conducted an in-depth analysis of the cause of the mistake and uncovered fifty separate failures in the hospital that contributed to the error. If any one of these failures had been detected, the infant would not have suffered harm. Some of the failures included a drug order—handwritten by a physician—that was unclear; a pharmacist who filled the order with a tenfold overdose; and the absence of a warning system to alert the pharmacist to the overdose.

After hearing the analysis, and after only forty-five minutes of delib-
erations, the jury found the nurse on trial not guilty. More than that, the
jurors demonstrated their personal support for the nurse by tearfully hug-
ging her after they rendered their verdict. They recognized that the nurse
was not to blame, because she was working in an organization whose
management did not put systems in place that could have prevented the
chain of mistakes that led to the tragic error.[21]

Obviously healthcare is a dangerous, complex, and complicated
industry, so it usually takes time to reconstruct a case in order to understand what happened from the point of view of those who were
involved in it. A rush to judgment is likely to precipitate more unnecessary harm. Moreover, as explained by Malcolm Gladwell in *Outliers*,
at least seven consecutive errors typically occur before culminating in
a serious safety event.[22]

ACCIDENTS, MISTAKES, AND FAILURES

There are legitimate instances of negligence that warrant punishment.
For example, I was recently involved with a case of psychiatrists who
kept prescribing Adderall—a highly addictive stimulant drug—to an
aspiring medical student who had clearly become addicted to the drug.
As reported by *The New York Times* in a front-page story about Richard
Fee, one of the psychiatrists even continued to prescribe Adderall after
Richard had been hospitalized for his addiction to the drug and after
his parents showed up to personally warn the psychiatrist that their son
would die if he continued to receive Adderall prescriptions. Part of the
problem was that the psychiatrist was prescribing the medication at a
dose that was higher than the maximum recommended dosage.[23] To
make matters worse, Richard clearly never had the condition for which
the drug was being prescribed—ADHD. There were so many egregious
errors in Richard's care, and failed opportunities to rely on established
safeguards, that the Virginia Board of Medicine recognized the psychiatrist's negligence and he was put out of practice.[24] When it comes to
patient safety events, such obvious and blatant negligence is the exception, not the rule. (Sadly, misdiagnosis and unwarranted medicalization
of everyday life struggles continue to plague the mental health field.)

As Megan McArdle explains in *The Up Side of Down*, there are important distinctions between accidents, mistakes, and failures. Such distinctions can prove to be significant when considering culpability, compensation, and punishment. An *accident* involves a situation "that could not have been plausibly expected or planned for" with this hallmark sign:

> While there may be lots of things you could have done differently, there is absolutely nothing you should have done differently. Aside from perfect foresight, there is no hard-won knowledge that you wish you could have applied, no error in judgment that can inform your decisions in the future.[25]

Sometimes accidents turn out all right, sometimes they don't. As an example of an accident that didn't end in disaster, McArdle describes a car crash that a friend experienced with a rental car. The car was rented from a reputable company, and there was no driver error involved in the accident. However, the steering system failed without warning, causing the vehicle to careen out of control and sending five cars flying across the highway. By an apparent miracle, McArdle's friend was essentially unharmed.

Just like that car accident, genuine unforeseen complications can happen during the delivery of clinical care. For example, when a patient has a severe first-time allergic reaction to medication during a surgical procedure, things can spin out of control (much like the rental car). Provided that the appropriate recovery medications are on hand, things might turn out okay. However, if the patient's medical status was compromised before surgery, the unforeseeable allergic reaction could precipitate complications from which the patient might not be able to recover. Yet even if the patient were to die, no error—just unpreventable complications—would have occurred.

A *mistake* is practically the opposite of an accident:

> It's where you could and maybe should have done something differently, but nothing really bad happens as a result. You spell *embarrass* wrong and the spell-checker corrects it before you're finished typing. You enter the wrong number into the budget spreadsheet, and then have to spend your lunch hour hunting down the discrepancy. You forget the grocery list and

come home with wine instead of the milk your spouse wanted. Most mistakes are trivial. But even big mistakes usually turn out all right.[26]

A mistake is when a doctor or nurse forgets to wash their hands but no harm comes of it in that particular instance; it is when a nurse gives Tylenol to the wrong patient without realizing it and without causing harm to anybody; or when my physical therapist initially treated the wrong leg. In each case, there were things that could have and should have been done differently or done better to avoid the mistakes.

Think back to Josie's story in chapter 5. The first time Josie needed naloxone as a rescue drug, one could argue that mistakes had been made—she was prescribed too much pain medication relative to her medical status, and she was not monitored closely enough. Even so, things turned out all right that first time. But when Josie was oversedated a second time, the story was altogether different. A series of errors snowballed (holes in the proverbial Swiss cheese lined up), and Josie was oversedated beyond the point of recovery. This was an instance of a failure—a catastrophic event that culminated from a series of mistakes. As McArdle describes it, a *failure* is "a mistake performing without a safety net." Said another way, failure occurs when:

> The fail-safes aren't failing safely any more. Suddenly, something has gone terribly wrong, and worse, if someone had only done things differently— better—it could have been prevented.[27]

McArdle goes on to describe her mother's hospital experience of having a ruptured appendix misdiagnosed. There were a number of small errors in judgment, "simple things, but each error made the other ones more dangerous, like sticks of kindling to a roaring fire."[28] Unfortunately, the person who commits that last in a series of errors, or the error that is most immediately evident, is often blamed for the whole cascading debacle. Upon further review, this person is typically found to be only partially to blame and sometimes to be entirely blame-free by virtue of having been set up for error by defects in broader system or workflow processes.

Sometimes a devastatingly poor outcome can occur in the hands of knowledgeable and caring providers because what transpires at the "sharp end of care" (at the bedside, so to speak) is affected by decisions that are made and policies that are developed at the "blunt end of care" (in the board room and executive offices). Exactly as the Swiss Cheese Model predicts, a wide range of blunt end (system) factors can determine the likelihood of a catastrophic failure. Notable among harm-inducing blunt end factors are inadequate staffing and training; unrealistic reliance on technology; and toxic working environments where people are threatened, bullied, or intimidated if they speak up about safety.

When researchers looked at nurse staffing levels and outcomes among surgical patients in two hospitals for an entire year, they discovered that every patient added to a nurse's caseload resulted in a 7 percent increase in patient deaths during hospitalization. Each additional patient added another 7 percent increase in patient deaths within thirty days of being discharged from the hospital.[29] Research has also documented a direct and sizable link between nurse-patient staffing ratios and medication errors.[30] Likewise, the less favorable the patient-nursing ratio, the longer patients need to be hospitalized,[31] which, in turn, increases the odds that they will suffer from healthcare-induced harm. Even the degree of disrespectful communication among staff members affects patient outcomes and survival rates.

Although system issues affect the frequency of human error and the likelihood of catastrophic failure, sadly, we tend to disregard or devalue these facts. Far too often, people respond by blaming and shaming the "last man standing." The impulse to seek others to blame is not without cause. It wasn't too many years ago when a hospital CEO told one of the authors of *Wall of Silence* that the way he tracked patient safety events was by nurse firings—every time a nurse was fired, he knew there had been an incident. In a few cases, public rallying cries have emerged in an effort to protect providers who have been judged too harshly.[32] More typically, though, providers suffer in isolation, which undoubtedly contributes to many providers changing jobs or leaving the profession.[33]

CULTURE TRUMPS POLICY

In addition to feeling guilty and ashamed about having one's errors exposed, physicians worry considerably about being sued. It is difficult to gather comprehensive information about the number of malpractice claims filed each year because there is no universal tracking system. However, a large-scale study in the *New England Journal of Medicine* estimated that 75 percent of US physicians in low-risk specialties and 99 percent of them in high-risk specialties could expect to face a malpractice claim during the course of their careers. When surveyed, 5 percent of physicians indicated that they had faced a malpractice claim within the previous year.[34] One objective source indicated that for each year between 1991 and 2005, over 7 percent of physicians had a malpractice claim filed against them with close to 20 percent resulting in a payment—a rate that is just slightly higher than the self-reported rate.[35]

For over one hundred years, the code of medical ethics has demanded that physicians self-report malpractice claims against them, but, on the whole, physicians have ignored this standard. Moreover, in most states, American physicians are not legally compelled to disclose malpractice to their patients. To address the gap between ethical and legal obligations, as of 2001 the Joint Commission began requiring that hospitals have policies that support the disclosure of adverse outcomes. Accordingly, *full disclosure* refers to:

> Communication of a healthcare provider and a patient, family member, or the patient's proxy that acknowledges the occurrence of an error, discusses what happened, and describes the link between the error and outcomes in a manner that is meaningful to the patient.[36]

Gradually, hospitals began writing policies to support the concept of full disclosure. Ironically, as the table below suggests, full-disclosure practices stand to benefit everyone, not just patients. The process breaks down the wall of silence and secrecy that interferes with opportunities for all parties to identify mistakes, fix causes of error, and heal. Nonetheless, the knee-jerk reaction of most physicians and hospitals continues to be to deny culpability.[37]

Some studies suggest that physicians disclose errors to patients only 25 percent to 30 percent of the times required by ethical standards and policy.[38] More recent evidence from one of the largest US healthcare systems suggests that full disclosure may be practiced much less often—even if full-disclosure policies are well publicized.[39] Most phy-

Table 7.1.

Responding to Medical Mistakes		
Impact	Typical Reaction	Full Disclosure
Patients and Families	• Blame the "last man standing" • Threaten legal action • Cut off contact with providers	• Reduce anger, support the grieving process • Ask questions, expect answers • Participate in the investigation, if desired • Foster healing and opportunities for forgiveness
Providers	• Feel guilty, lose confidence and joy • Deny error, blame others • Avoid patient and family	• Seek emotional support • Communicate openly with patient • Apologize to patients, families, and coworkers • Recover sense of confidence and joy
Hospitals	• Sweep errors under the rug • Limit contact with family • Avoid all liability	• Apologize to patient and family • Investigate the event thoroughly • Invite patients to contribute to inquiry • Accept responsibility, as appropriate • Deny culpability, as appropriate • Resolve legal issues in a timely fashion • Tend to emotional needs of staff • Find and fix causes of error • Share lessons learned • Create safer facilities and providers
Society	• Undermines Progress and Healing	• Safeguards People and Institutions

sicians and hospitals still do not disclose medical errors unless forced to do so,[40] but even then they tend do so ineffectively.[41] When confronted with hypothetical cases, physician responses included instances of partial disclosure that often made it difficult to connect provider error to the adverse outcome.[42]

Why, in spite of requirements that direct physicians to speak openly and plainly about medical errors, does full disclosure occur so infrequently? In addition to fears of litigation and reputation loss, physicians are subjected to a hidden curriculum that trains them to bury their mistakes. The *hidden curriculum* refers to:

> The messages transmitted implicitly on the job, through everyday vocabulary, practices, and habits, all of which have powerful effects on individual attitudes and practices. This phenomenon is particularly relevant to medicine, where longstanding, and often rigid, traditions about hierarchy allow actions of senior physicians—positive and negative—to strongly influence student behavior.[43]

THE SHAME THAT DIVIDES US

The book *Wall of Silence* describes what seems like countless, horrific stories of hospital errors. In one chapter alone, they describe ten patient safety cases, which are summarized below.

Many Faces of Healthcare-Induced Harm

- World War II veteran: Okie was a strong and energetic husband and father to four children, but he died because a nurse failed to attend to a written order stating not to reinsert the tube that passed from his nose to his stomach if it came out.
- White House executive: Daniel underwent what turned out to be an unnecessary surgery that caused cranial nerve damage, leaving him debilitated and unemployed in the prime of his life.
- Emmy Award–winning TV news anchor: Mary underwent cosmetic surgery to maintain her TV ratings, but she was left with pain that is so debilitating she is unable to work or socialize normally.
- Wise beyond her years: Eight-year-old Elizabeth is permanently paralyzed from the waist down because doctors didn't listen when she told them her cancer was back. As she lay suffering, the sensitive young girl wanted to know why the doctors didn't believe her.
- Financial manager: Susan suffered a botched laparoscopic procedure, required multiple follow-up surgeries, $150,000 in medical bills that weren't covered by insurance, and lifelong pain and difficulty going to the bathroom.

- Mother and real estate agent: Marion was an optimistic and cheerful woman who died while waiting for her first cancer treatment because the staff oversedated her with opiate pain medication that she didn't need or request.
- Former Air Force intelligence officer: Diana was in her thirties and in good shape. She worked out regularly despite ongoing hip pain. After much debate, she elected to undergo a surgical procedure to correct the situation. The surgery went well, but Diana was left unattended for hours and unable to get any medical attention. Outraged by poor postoperative care, she transferred to another hospital. While still weak and "fuzzy" from the surgery and drugs, she fell. Her pain worsened, but she was written off as "hypersensitive" and her pain medications were increased. It turns out that her new joint had been dislocated. Because the dislocated hip was overlooked for weeks, Diana needed several more surgeries, which were also error-ridden experiences, and it was years before all the damage from the initial postoperative failures were resolved.
- Model high school student: In so many ways, fifteen-year-old Lewis was every parent's dream child. He was admitted for surgery to undergo a new procedure for fixing a relatively common sunken chest condition called *pectus excavatum*. The new surgical procedure was a success, but Lewis died because he developed a bleeding ulcer from a powerful painkiller and the hospital nurses repeatedly disregarded his complaints and alarming symptoms.
- Grandmother with a will to live: Madeline lost twenty-five pounds and deteriorated rapidly from severe pain due to staff failure to address her complaints—described like a knife in her side—or to notice that an X-ray clearly showed that a four-inch pin used to hold broken bones in place had come loose and traveled into surrounding hip tissue. She needed additional surgery, and it took three years for her to regain her strength.
- Star quarterback and college student: Justin was a healthy and tough young man, but he died within two days of visiting a hospital where a serious infection was overlooked in spite of signs that septic shock was setting in.

What do these seemingly diverse patient safety stories have in common? Nobody who cared for these patients ever apologized for the mistakes that occurred—except one of the many physicians who treated all the patients harmed. Imagine you were Elizabeth's mother and that as she lay there learning to cope with a life of paralysis, her request to meet with her doctors to ask, "Why didn't you believe me?" was repeatedly denied. If that isn't a case of unnecessary pain being inflicted on a traumatized girl and her mother, I don't know what is. And yet, here's what the young girl said to her distraught mother, "I forgive you, Mom, but you have to forgive yourself."[44]

Time and again, the victims profiled in *Wall of Silence* expressed the sentiment that they could live with the mistakes that were made, but not with the fact that nobody would apologize for them. As Okie's wife said, "We need hospitals to speak up and tell the family that a mistake was made and consult with them to explain what happened. This would have meant a great deal to me and helped in the healing process."[45] And here's how a woman whose father died because his blood thinner was refilled incorrectly explained the need for an apology.

Adding Insult to Injury

Just think if my neighbor is driving down the road in front of my house, and I'm looking out my window and see him hit my dog that was running across the street. If he gets out of his car and picks up my dog and brings him up to the house, truly sad and upset for what happened, how can I be mad at him? I would try to make him feel not so bad for something he certainly didn't intend to do. But if he kept on driving and later comes up to the house, lies to me, and says he didn't do it, and yet I saw him do it, you can imagine how mad that would make me feel.[46]

IT'S NOT ALL ABOUT PHYSICIANS

What is also disconcerting about current disclosure practices is that nurses, pharmacists, respiratory therapists, physical therapists, and all other healthcare workers have been largely omitted from the discussion about how to handle the aftermath of medical errors, even when they have been directly involved in them. Given nurses' central role in the care of patients, this is a particularly significant oversight. The

American Association of Colleges of Nursing describes the role of nursing this way:

> Though often working collaboratively, nursing does not "assist" medicine or other fields. Nursing operates independent of, not auxiliary to, medicine and other disciplines. Nurses' roles range from direct patient care and case management to establishing nursing practice standards, developing quality assurance procedures, and directing complex nursing care systems.[47]

And yet, when it comes to disclosure, typically nurses have been treated as a dyad wherein the physician and/or hospital can plan for disclosure and communicate with patients without their input or involvement. Not surprisingly, some nurses report being left in ethically compromising positions, sometimes feeling the need to disclose errors to patients without physician awareness.[48] Like physicians, nurses (and all licensed providers) can be sued.[49]

Excluding any member of the healthcare team, preventing them from honestly and appropriately disclosing errors, or confronting them with undue criticism or punishment can exacerbate their stress. High stress leads to underperformance and burnout that, in turn, increases the likelihood the providers will become more error-prone.

OPENNESS AND HEALING

Hiding mistakes not only adds insult to injury for patients and families, it also complicates and compromises the healing and learning of providers. Again, in the words of Dr. Wu:

Guilt, Confession, and Recovery

> It has been suggested that the only way to face the guilt after a serious error is through confession, restitution, and absolution. But confession is discouraged, passively by the lack of appropriate forums for discussion, and sometimes actively by risk managers and hospital lawyers. . . .
>
> In the absence of mechanisms for healing, physicians find dysfunctional ways to protect themselves . . . Distress escalates in the face of a malpractice suit. In the long run, some physicians are deeply wounded, lose their nerve, burn out, or seek solace in alcohol or drugs.[50]

Fortunately for all of us, in the wake of Josie King's death in 2001, Johns Hopkins took the bold step of becoming the first hospital to openly disclose what went wrong with the family, invited the family to be part of the investigation, and shared the lessons learned with the hospital community and broader public. Although Sorrel King and her husband, Tony, elected not to participate in the investigation, the hospital kept them abreast of everything that was learned. A hospital executive gave Sorrel his direct phone number with an invitation to call at any time, and he set up a weekly conference call to share with her the progress of the investigation.[51]

Such openness is critical because the investigation of a patient safety event can take weeks or months to complete and asking patients to wait until the process is over for any feedback is inhumane. Excluding patients from knowing what is going on behind the scenes can worsen their fears and doubts, engendering a greater sense of distrust and anger. In fact, nearly half of malpractice claims are filed because patients and families had become suspicious that providers were covering up mistakes or because they wanted information.[52]

Wu and others from Johns Hopkins now advise healthcare institutions and train providers to treat disclosure as part of the ongoing dialogue with the patient and/or the patient's family. They believe that keeping patients and families informed about everything as it is being learned is simply a matter of providing decent, quality care. It is also consistent with the modern healthcare notion of "nothing about me without me." As full disclosure champions, Wu and his colleagues speak about the "golden hour" for sharing information with patients. They recognize that failure to be immediately forthcoming can break trust when disclosure finally occurs, creating the worrisome sense of, "You mean, you knew this all along and weren't telling me?"[53] Although there is a long way to go before full disclosure becomes a routine practice, there is evidence that people have been listening.

In 2000, only 29 percent of first-year medical residents indicated that they would disclose a medical error to patients; by 2009, the number was up to 55 percent.[54] The number of hospitals that have implemented full-disclosure policies also continues to rise. A critical lesson that has been learned from trailblazing institutions such as Johns Hopkins, the VA Health Care System in Louisville, Kentucky, the Michigan Health System, and Ascension Health as well as from efforts to replicate their efforts is this: the success of full-disclosure policies depends on the organizational culture in which they are embedded.[55] And the great news is that with sufficient preparation, internal promotion, and professional training, full-disclosure programs can work incredibly well.[56]

Ascension Health—a large healthcare system with over seventy hospitals and hundreds of outpatient facilities in at least half the United States—provides one of the most recent and compelling stories of the power of a strategically implemented full-disclosure program. In 2007, Ascension implemented a full-disclosure policy across its system with the goal of 100 percent adoption, but it turned out that only about 10 percent of hospital teams and providers adhered to the policy. Culture trumped policy, just as it did with the Rhode Island hospital described in chapter 4. So, in 2011, Ascension transformed its policy into a manageable program—a program that is consistent with the elements that have become recognized as essential to effective disclosure.[57]

Leaders selected a handful of labor and delivery sites to develop, implement, and evaluate the process. First, program leaders created a single and easily understood protocol out of the existing protocols that varied in length and clarity. They also held meetings to introduce the program before expecting compliance, trained a response team at each hospital to facilitate and be accountable for the process, and provided each hospital with disclosure coaches who had been prepared to assist providers and administrators when events occurred. Ascension also collaborated with a medical liability insurance company to develop and provide physicians premium credit for completing error analysis and disclosure training. Their strategic efforts to translate policy into action paid off.

Twelve months into the program, 43 percent of participants supported full disclosure; after twenty-seven months, 77 percent fully supported it. What's more, by about two years into the program, participant buy-in was accompanied by a 221 percent increase in the rate of documented disclosures across all participating facilities.[58]

Ascension used scripts to train providers on what to say when discussing adverse outcomes with patients in a manner that would attend to all the elements that Wu and colleagues have identified as essential to effective disclosure.[59] As the table below suggests, the concept of full disclosure is intended to meet the needs of patients and families, but each element also confers potential benefits to healthcare providers.

Table 7.2.

Key Elements of Full Disclosure		
Key Elements	**What Patients Desire**	**Potential Benefit to Providers**
Explanation	Timely accounting of what went wrong and why it happened	Maintain patient's trust, improve safety knowledge
Responsibility	Appropriate ownership by provider and/or hospital for what went wrong	Reduce likelihood of a lawsuit
Apology	Sincere apology with expression of provider's distress and sympathy for patient or family	Experience emotional relief, lessen likelihood of second victim phenomenon
Prevention	Promise effort will be made to learn from the event and prevent similar recurrences	Strengthen and reinforce a culture of safety
Compensation	Nonadversarial process to ensure financial reparations	Hasten resolution and healing, decrease litigation and settlement time and costs

The Ascension program relied on highly scripted language that employees practiced in advance of disclosing information about adverse outcomes to patients, which the staff reported was very helpful. These scripts represent not only what providers need to learn to say, they are also what patients need to hear. In addition to modeling how to translate hospital policy into action, the Ascension story can serve as a blueprint of how a community coalition might implement changes it prioritizes.

Disclosing Potential Error[60]

We are sorry that this event occurred and want you to know it is being reviewed carefully to determine the cause. As soon as this assessment is completed, we will meet with you to let you know the findings.[61]

Disclosing an Error-Free Adverse Event

We are very sorry that this event has occurred. We have completed the review and the event was not preventable for the following reasons.[62]

Disclosing Healthcare-Induced Harm

We are very sorry that our actions led to this very disappointing outcome. We would like to explain what happened and what changes we have made so this won't happen again. We will work with you to try to make you whole and earn back your trust.[63]

As the public becomes more aware of the nature of the patient safety crisis, we cannot afford to delay the educational reforms that are necessary to support full disclosure or to neglect the needs of providers who are honest with their patients. Fortunately, over thirty states have laws in place to protect physician apologies from liability, recognizing that apologizing does not necessarily imply guilt.[64] In time, the public may gain appreciation for the fact that sometimes patients deserve to be compensated without meaning that the provider deserves to be punished.

THE ECONOMICS OF HONESTY

Being honest and transparent with patients about medical errors is not only the right thing to do, it also pays dividends. In 2001, the University of Michigan Health System began fully disclosing medical errors to patients and families and offering them compensation for such errors. An analysis of claims data for six years before and six years after the system began fully disclosing medical errors provided substantial evidence of the financial benefit of being honest and transparent with patients and their attorneys. After the disclosure program began, the average rate of new claims fell by 36 percent. The average monthly rate of lawsuits also decreased by 65 percent. The median time from claim reporting to resolution was shortened by 30 percent. The healthcare system's average monthly cost rate for total liability, patient compensation, and noncompensation-related legal costs all decreased by about 40 percent.[65]

In 2009, the Agency for Healthcare Research and Quality dispersed $25 million to support demonstration projects related to full disclosure and medical liability reform, including the Ascension program.[66] These projects suggest there is still much to be learned about the best ways to connect full-disclosure communications with compensation mechanisms and models. It is possible that disclosing errors and offering compensation before a malpractice claim is filed may lead to an in-crease in the number of claims filed.[67] Even so, this practice could still be beneficial to patients without having a negative impact on the bot-tom line of institutions or insurance providers because about 85 percent do not merit compensation[68] and the majority of medical malpractice dollars are spent on legal fees (not on victim compensation or punitive damages).[69] Furthermore, the process is more conducive to learning and healing from adverse events and to preventing their recurrence.

In the words of a public health professional, an attorney, and a physician:

> Ultimately we cannot deliver the safest possible care unless we foster an environment in which healthcare workers have a safe place to grapple with the impact of their involvement in adverse events. If our legal struc-tures create a chilling effect on these communications, then healthcare professionals, patients, and the system as a whole suffer in the long run.[70]

UNITED, WE ALL GAIN

Just think of the agony and cost to patients, providers, institutions, and society that could be averted through greater openness about medical mistakes. As Gorovitz and MacIntyre noted four decades ago:

> It follows that injury is no proof of culpability. If physicians were to act as if they recognized this point, they might become far less reluctant to acknowledge, systematize, and learn from injury. But that would require a widespread willingness on the part of patients also to acknowledge this point, and thereby lower their expectations about what physicians can accomplish, and to refrain from assuming, even in the disappointment or despair that attends iatrogenic [healthcare-induced] injury, that the physician is culpable.[71]

We truly are in this together. The sooner we accept the imperfect nature of healthcare and apologize for mistakes when they do occur, the more we will learn from our mistakes and the quicker and better we will recover from the physical, emotional, financial, and societal wounds that medical errors can cause. In the words of Alexander Pope, a seventeenth-century poet: "To err is human; to forgive, divine."

Notes

CHAPTER 1

1. Donald M. Berwick, 2016. Permission granted via November 15, 2016, email from Donald Berwick to ascribe this quote to him.

2. Alan L. Mackay, *A Dictionary of Scientific Quotations* (Bristol, UK: Institute of Physics Publishing, 1991).

3. J. T. James, "A New, Evidence-Based Estimate of Patient Harms Associated with Hospital Care," *Journal of Patient Safety* 9, no. 3 (2013).

4. Martin A. Makary and Michael Daniel, "Medical Error—the Third Leading Cause of Death in the US," *BMJ* 353 (2016).

5. L. Binder, "Stunning News on Preventable Deaths in Hospitals," *Forbes Magazine*, September 23, 2013, http://www.forbes.com/sites/leah binder/2013/09/23/stunning-news-on-preventable-deaths-in-hospitals/.

6. L. L. Leape et al., "Preventing Medical Injury," *Quarterly Review Bulletein* 19, no. 5 (1993).

7. R. Scott, "The Direct Medical Costs of Healthcare-Associated Infections in U.S. Hospitals and the Benefits of Prevention," ed. Centers for Disease Control and Prevention (CDC, 2009).

8. C. Andel et al., "The Economics of Health Care Quality and Medical Errors," *Journal of Health Care Finance* 39, no. 1 (2012).

9. D. C. Classen et al., "'Global Trigger Tool' Shows That Adverse Events in Hospitals May Be Ten Times Greater Than Previously Measured," *Health Affairs* 30, no. 4 (2011).

10. Judith H. Hibbard et al., "Can Patients Be Part of the Solution? Views on Their Role in Preventing Medical Errors," *Medical Care Research and Review* 62, no. 5 (2005).

11. E. G. Campbell et al., "Professionalism in Medicine: Results of a National Survey of Physicians," *Annals of Internal Medicine* 147, no. 11 (2007).

12. Institute of Medicine, *Patient Safety: Achieving a New Standard of Care* (Washington, DC: National Academies Press, 2004).

13. Campbell et al., "Professionalism in Medicine."

14. Occupational Safety and Health Administration, "Worker Safety in Your Hospital," https://www.osha.gov/dsg/hospitals/documents/1.1_Data_highlights_508.pdf.

15. James, "A New, Evidence-Based Estimate of Patient Harms Associated with Hospital Care."

16. Megan McArdle, *The Up Side of Down: Why Failing Well Is the Key to Success* (New York: Penquin Books, 2015).

17. J. M. Kane, M. Brannen, and E. Kern, "Impact of Patient Safety Mandates on Medical Education in the United States," *Journal of Patient Safety* 4, no. 2 (2008).

18. J. N. Deis et al., "Transforming the Morbidity and Mortality Conference into an Instrument for Systemwide Improvement," in *Advances in Patient Safety: New Directions and Alternative Approaches*, ed. K. Henriksen, J. B. Battles, and M. A. Keyes (Rockville, MD: Agency for Healthcare Research and Quality, 2008); Lucien Leape Institute, "Unmet Needs: Teaching Physicians to Provide Safe Patient Care" (Boston, MA: National Patient Safety Foundation, 2010).

19. L. T. Kohn, J. M. Corrigan, and M. S. Donaldson, *To Err Is Human: Building a Safer Health System* (Washington, DC: Institute of Medicine, 1999).

20. Kohn, Corrigan, and Donaldson, *To Err Is Human*.

21. L. L. Leape, "Scope of Problem and History of Patient Safety," *Obstetric and Gynecological Clinics of North America* 35 (2008).

22. Binder, "Stunning News on Preventable Deaths in Hospitals."

23. L. L. Leape and D. M. Berwick, "Five Years after *To Err Is Human*: What Have We Learned?" *JAMA* 293, no. 19 (2005).

24. G. H. Burke, G. B. LeFever, and S. M. Sayles, "Zero Events of Harm to Patients: Building and Sustaining a System-Wide Culture of Safety at Sentara Healthcare," *Managing Infection Control* (2009), http://www.yoursls.com/Culture-Safety-Healthcare.pdf.

25. R. Grol, D. M. Berwick, and M. Wensing, "On the Trail of Quality and Safety in Health Care," *BMJ: British Medical Journal* 336, no. 7635 (2008); K. Jewell and L. McGiffert, "To Err Is Human—to Delay Is Deadly: Ten Years Later, a Million Lives Lost, Billions of Dollars Wasted," *Consumers Union: Nonprofit Publishers of Consumer Reports* (2009), http://safepatient-project.org/pdf/safepatientproject.org.to_delay_is_deadly-2009_05.pdf.

26. D. Charles, M. Gabriel, and M. F. Furukawa, "Adoption of Electronic Health Record Systems among U.S. Non-Federal Acute Care Hospitals: 2008–2013," ONC, https://www.healthit.gov/sites/default/files/oncdatabrief16.pdf.

27. William F. Bria, "The Electronic Health Record: Is It Meaningful Yet?" *Mayo Clinic Proceedings* 86, no. 5 (2011); D. F. Carr, "Electronic Health Records: First, Do No Harm?" *InformationWeek* (2014), http://www.informationweek.com/healthcare/electronic-health-records/electronic-health-records-first-do-no-harm/a/d-id/1278834; J. Sidorov, "It Ain't Necessarily So: The Electronic Health Record and the Unlikely Prospect of Reducing Health Care Costs: Much of the Literature on Ehrs Fails to Support the Primary Rationales for Using Them," *Health Affairs* 25, no. 4 (2006).

28. Stacy Parker, "Health Care Hero Awards: Corporate Achievements in Health Care," *Inside Business*, February 17, 2012; Robert Wachter, *The Digital Doctor: Hope, Hype, and Harm at the Dawn of Medicine's Computer Age* (New York: McGraw-Hill, 2015).

29. Wachter, *The Digital Doctor*.

30. M. R. Chassin and J. M. Loeb, "High-Reliability Health Care: Getting There from Here," *Milbank Quarterly* 91, no. 3 (2013).

31. R. M. Wachter to Wachter's World, February 18, 2013, http://blogs.hospitalmedicine.org/Blog/is-the-patient-safety-movement-in-danger-of-flickering-out/ http://community.the-hospitalist.org/2013/02/18/is-the-patient-safety-movement-in-danger-of-flickering-out/.

32. Wachter's World.

33. Comment regarding Denham: I experienced the same ingratiating treatment in 2013 when Denham was interested in connecting with the $16 million HITECH grant that I was directing for the purpose of establishing leadership training for healthcare professionals involved with implementing new technology in their facilities. To this day, it is disconcerting to look back and wonder whether his motives were pure. In spite of his acts of impropriety, Denham did make positive and lasting contributions to the field of patient safety.

34. G. L. Watson, "The Hospital Safety Crisis: Unifying Efforts of Healthcare Systems, Public Health, and Society," *Society* 53, no. 4 (2016).

35. Hibbard et al., "Can Patients Be Part of the Solution?"

36. Comment regarding off-the-mark procedure terminology: off-the-mark procedures refer to what the field typically calls wrong-site surgeries. For reasons explained in chapter 5, use of the term *off-the-mark procedures* eliminates the considerable confusion that has stemmed from the use of the term *wrong-site surgeries*.

37. Comment regarding frequency of off-the-mark procedures: although off-the-mark procedures occur much less often than healthcare-associated

infections and medication errors, this is one of the most preventable types of medical error. All three types of error can be prevented with consistent use of specific behaviors that laypersons could and should learn to observe and/or request. Together, they comprise as much as half of all medical errors.

CHAPTER 2

1. Comment regarding Lucien Leape quote: Countless presentations and articles ascribe this quote to Dr. Lucien L. Leape, a physician at Harvard School of Public Health who has been a leader of the patient safety movement. I have not been able to document the original source, but I have requested permission to ascribe this quote to Dr. Leape.

2. Leah Binder, "The Leapfrog Annual Hospital Survey," personal communication email, 2013.

3. Leah Binder and William H. Finck, "Results of the 2013 Leapfrog Hospital Survey: Executive Summary," 2015, http://www.leapfroggroup.org/sites/default/files/Files/2013LeapfrogHospitalSurveyResultsReport.pdf.

4. Centers for Disease Control and Prevention, "General Information about MRSA in the Community," Centers for Disease Control and Prevention.

5. James Reason, "Human Error: Models and Management," *BMJ: British Medical Journal* 320, no. 7237 (2000).

6. C. Duhigg, *The Power of Habit: Why We Do What We Do in Life and Business* (New York: Random House, 2014).

7. G. Rubin, *Better Than Before: Mastering the Habits of Our Everyday Lives* (New York: Crown Publishers, 2015).

8. Gordon Kraft-Todd et al., "Promoting Cooperation in the Field," *Current Opinion in Behavioral Sciences* 3 (2015).

9. Jennifer Jacquet, *Is Shame Necessary?: New Uses for an Old Tool* (New York: Random House, 2015).

10. Jacquet, *Is Shame Necessary?* 173.

11. Josep Call et al., "Domestic Dogs (Canis Familiaris) Are Sensitive to the Attentional State of Humans," *Comparative Psychology* 117, no. 3 (2003).

12. J. H. Hibbard, J. Stockard, and M. Tusler, "Does Publicizing Hospital Performance Stimulate Quality Improvement Efforts?" *Health Affairs* 22, no. 2 (2003).

13. I. M. Rosenstock, V. J. Stretcher, and M. H. Becker, "Social Learning Theory and the Health Belief Model," *Health Education Quarterly* 15, no. 2 (1988).

14. S. B. Fawcett et al., "Using Empowerment Theory in Collaborative Partnership for Community Health and Development," *American Journal of Community Psychology* 23, no. 5 (1995); D. J. McCloskey et al., "Community Engagement: Definitions and Organizing Concepts from the Literature," ed. Public Health Practice Program Office (Atlanta, GA: Centers for Disease Control and Prevention, 2015).

15. Angela Coulter and Jo Ellins, "Effectiveness of Strategies for Informing, Educating, and Involving Patients," *BMJ: British Medical Journal* 335, no. 7609 (2007).

16. Donald M. Berwick, "What 'Patient-Centered' Should Mean: Confessions of an Extremist," *Health Affairs* 28, no. 4 (2009).

17. Center for Advancing Health, "A New Definition of Patient Engagement: What Is Engagement and Why Is It Important?" (Washington DC: 2010).

18. Audrey Revere, "JCAHO National Patient Safety Goals for 2007," *Topics in Patient Safety* 7, no. 1 (2007), VA National Center for Patient Safety.

19. Coulter and Ellins, "Effectiveness of Strategies for Informing, Educating, and Involving Patients."

20. Amy D. Waterman et al., "Brief Report: Hospitalized Patients' Attitudes About and Participation in Error Prevention," *Journal of General Internal Medicine* 21, no. 4 (2006).

21. M. McGuckin et al., "Evaluation of a Patient-Empowering Hand Hygiene Programme in the UK," *Journal of Hospital Infection* 48, no. 3 (2001).

22. Christopher Paul Duncan and Carol Dealey, "Patients' Feelings About Hand Washing, MRSA Status and Patient Information," *British Journal of Nursing* 16, no. 1 (2007).

23. Monash Institute of Health Service Research, "Literature Review Regarding Patient Engagement in Patient Safety Initiatives," 2008, http://www.safetyandquality.gov.au/wp-content/uploads/2012/01/Literature-Review-Regarding-Patient-Engagement-in-Patient-Safety-Initiatives.pdf.

24. Maureen Maurer et al., "Guide to Parent and Family Engagement: Environmental Scan Report," in *AHRQ Publication No. 12-0042-EF* (Rockville, MD: Agency for Healthcare Research and Quality, 2012).

25. Maurer et al., "Guide to Parent and Family Engagement."

26. M. K. Paasche-Orlow et al., "The Prevalence of Limited Health Literacy," *Journal of General Internal Medicine* 20, no. 2 (2005).

27. Vikki Entwistle, Michelle M. Mello, and Troyen A. Brennan, "Advising Patients About Patient Safety: Current Initiatives Risk Shifting Responsibility," *Journal on Quality and Patient Safety* 31, no. 9 (2005).

28. National Patient Safety Foundation, "Health Literacy: Statistics at-a-Glance," 2011, https://c.ymcdn.com/sites/www.npsf.org/resource/collec tion/9220B314-9666-40DA-89DA-9F46357530F1/AskMe3_Stats_English.pdf.

29. Cecelia Conrath Doak, Leonard G. Doak, and Jane H. Root, "The Literacy Problem," in *Teaching Patients with Low Literacy Skills* (Philadelphia: J. B. Lippincott Co., 1996).

30. Irwin S. Kirsch et al., "Adult Literacy in America: A First Look at the Findings of the National Adult Literacy Survey," ed. Office of Educational Research and Improvement (U.S. Department of Education, 2002).

31. Paasche-Orlow et al., "The Prevalence of Limited Health Literacy."

32. Doak, Doak, and Root, "The Literacy Problem."

33. Maurer et al., "Guide to Parent and Family Engagement," 2.

34. Vikki Entwistle, "Nursing Shortages and Patient Safety Problems in the Hospital Care: Is Clinical Monitoring by Families Part of the Solution?" *Health Expectations* 7 (2004); Entwistle, Mello, and Brennan, "Advising Patients About Patient Safety."

35. G. B. LeFever, "Chasing Zero Events of Harm: An Urgent Call to Expand Safety Culture Work and Patient Engagement," *Nursing and Patient Care* (February 2010), http://www.yoursls.com/ConnectingHospitals-Communities.pdf.

36. M. Leonard, S. Graham, and D. Bonacum, "The Human Factor: The Critical Importance of Effective Teamwork and Communication in Providing Safe Care," *Quality and Safety in Health Care* 13, no. Suppl. 1 (2004).

37. J. Sorra et al., "Hospital Survey on Patient Safety Culture" (Rockville, MD: Agency for Healthcare Research and Quality, 2012).

38. Ayako Okuyama, Cordula Wagner, and Bart Bijnen, "Speaking up for Patient Safety by Hospital-Based Health Care Professionals: A Literature Review," *BMC Health Services Research* 14 (2014).

39. M. J. Bittle and S. LaMarch, "Engaging the Patient as Observer to Promote Hand Hygiene Compliance in Ambulatory Care," *The Joint Commission Journal on Quality and Patient Safety* 35, no. 10 (2009).

40. Comment on the Joint Commission's Center for Transforming Healthcare: The Joint Commission formed the Center for Transforming Healthcare in 2008 to solve healthcare's most pressing issues. Eliminating healthcare-associated infections has been one of its primary initiatives (http://www.centerfortransforminghealthcare.org).

41. Duhigg, *The Power of Habit*.

CHAPTER 3

1. Sanjaya Kumar, *Fatal Care: Survive in the U.S. Health System* (Minneapolis, MN: IGI Press, 2008).

2. Infection Control Today, "Hospitals Pair Germ-Killing Robots with CDC Protocols to Protect against Ebola Virus," *Infection Control Today* (2014), http://www.infectioncontroltoday.com/news/2014/10/hospitals-pair -germkilling-robots-with-cdc-protocols-to-protect-against-ebola-virus.aspx.

3. G. B. LeFever, "Chasing Zero Events of Harm: An Urgent Call to Expand Safety Culture Work and Patient Engagement," *Nursing and Patient Care* (February 2010), http://www.yoursls.com/ConnectingHospitals-Com munities.pdf.

4. World Health Organization, *WHO Guidelines on Hand Hygiene in Health Care: A Summary* (Geneva, Switzerland: World Health Organization, 2009).

5. K. L. Cummings, D. J. Anderson, and K. S. Kaye, "Hand Hygiene Noncompliance and the Cost of Hospital-Acquired Methicillin-Resistant Staphylococcus Aureus Infection," *Infection Control and Hospital Epidemiology* 31, no. 4 (2010): 357–64.

6. K. Sack, "A Hospital Hand-Washing Project to Save Lives and Money," *New York Times*, September 10, 2009.

7. Stephen Y. Liang, Daniel L. Theodoro, Jeremiah D. Schuur, and Jonas Marschall, "Infection Prevention in the Emergency Department," *Infectious Disease* 64, no. 3 (2014): 299–313.

8. Randi Hutter Epstein, *Get Me Out: A History of Childbirth from the Garden of Eden to the Sperm Bank* (New York: W. W. Norton and Company, 2010).

9. C. R. Denham, P. Angood, D. Berwick, L. Binder, C. Clancy, J. Corrigan, and D. Hunt, "The Vital Link Department: Making Idealized Design a Reality," *Journal of Patient Safety* 5, no. 4 (2009): 216–22.

10. Charles R. Denham, Peter Angood, Don Berwick, Leah Binder, Carolyn M. Clancy, Janet M. Corrigan, and David Hunt, "Chasing Zero: Can Reality Meet the Rhetoric?" *Journal of Patient Safety* 5, no. 4 (2009): 216–22.

11. Frances S. Margolin, "Getting to Zero: Reducing Rates of CLABSI in Community Hospitals" (2011), http://haifocus.com/leapfrog-audio-replay-getting-to-zero-reducing-rates-of-clabsi-in-community-hospitals/.

12. Peter Pronovost, Dale Needham, Sean Berenholtz, David Sinopoli, Haitao Chu, Sara Cosgrove, Bryan Sexton et al., "An Intervention to Decrease Catheter-Related Bloodstream Infections in the ICU," *New England Journal of Medicine* 355, no. 26 (2006): 2725–32.

13. P. J. Pronovost and E. Vohr, *Safe Patients, Smart Hospitals: How One Doctor's Checklist Can Help Us Change Health Care from the Inside Out* (New York: Penquin Group, 2010).

14. Peter Pronovost, Christine A. Goeschel, Elizabeth Colantuoni, Sam Watson, Lisa H. Lubomski, Sean M. Berenholtz, David A. Thompson et al., "Sustaining Reductions in Catheter Related Bloodstream Infections in Michigan Intensive Care Units: Observational Study," *BMJ: British Medical Journal* 340 (2010): c309.

15. E. E. Sickbert-Bennett, L. M. Dibiase, W. Schade, E. S. Wolak, D. J. Weber, and W. A. Rutala, "Reduction of Healthcare-Associated Infections by Exceeding High Compliance with Hand Hygiene Practices," *Emerging Infectious Diseases* 22, no. 9 (2016): 1628–30.

16. Megan McArdle, *The Up Side of Down: Why Failing Well Is the Key to Success* (New York: Penquin Books, 2015).

17. McArdle, *The Up Side of Down*, 103.

18. R. M. Klevens, J. R. Edwards, C. L. Richards, T. C. Horan, R. P. Gaynes, D. A. Pollock, and D. M. Cardo, "Estimating Health Care-Associated Infections and Deaths in U.S. Hospitals, 2002," *Public Health Reports* 122 (2007): 160–66.

19. Chip Heath and Dan Heath, *Made to Stick: Why Some Ideas Survive and Others Die* (New York: Random House, 2007).

CHAPTER 4

1. Sanjaya Kumar, *Fatal Care: Survive in the U.S. Health System* (Minneapolis, MN: IGI Press, 2008).

2. John R. Clarke, Janet Johnston, and Edward D. Finley, "Getting Surgery Right," *Annals of Surgery* 246, no. 3 (2007).

3. Comment on never events: for a complete list of "never events," see http://psnet.ahrq.gov/resource.aspx?resourceID=3643.

4. Kim Smiley to Patient Safety Blog, January 16, 2014, http://www.patient -safety-blog.com/2014/01/16/the-willie-king-case-wrong-foot-amputated/.

5. Tatiana Morales, "Switched before Birth," 2004, http://www.cbsnews .com/news/switched-before-birth/.

6. J. Martinez, "What a Mess, Baby," *Daily News*, March 22, 2007.

7. Carol Kopp, "Anatomy of a Mistake," 2003, http://www.cbsnews.com/ news/anatomy-of-a-mistake-16-03-2003/.

8. David C. Ring, James H. Herndon, and Gregg S. Meyer, "Case 34-2010," *New England Journal of Medicine* 363, no. 20 (2010).

9. P. G. Shekelle et al., "Making Health Care Safer II: An Updated Critical Analysis of the Evidence for Patient Safety Practices," in *Comparative Effectiveness Review No. 211*, ed. Southern California-RAND Evidence-Based Practice Center (Rockville, MD: Agency for Healthcare Research and Quality, 2013).

10. P. F. Stahel et al., "Wrong-Site and Wrong-Patient Procedures in the Universal Protocol Era: Analysis of a Prospective Database of Physician Self-Reported Occurrences," *Archives of Surgery* 145, no. 10 (2010).

11. A. Gardner, "Surgery Mix-Ups Surprisingly Common," 2010, http://www.cnn.com/2010/HEALTH/10/18/health.surgery.mixups.common/.

12. P. J. Pronovost and E. Vohr, *Safe Patients, Smart Hospitals: How One Doctor's Checklist Can Help Us Change Health Care from the Inside Out* (New York: Penquin Group, 2010).

13. Thomas G. Weiser et al., "An Estimation of the Global Volume of Surgery: A Modelling Strategy Based on Available Data," *The Lancet* 372, no. 9633.

14. A. Gawande, *The Checklist Manifesto: How to Get Things Right* (New York: Metropolitan Books, 2009).

15. Associated Press, "Trail of Errors Led to 3 Wrong Brain Surgeries," 2007, http://www.nbcnews.com/id/22263412/ns/health-health_care/t/trail-errors-led-wrong-brain-surgeries/#.WBUSquErJTY.

16. "Trail of Errors Led to 3 Wrong Brain Surgeries: Surgeons' Ego at R.I. Hospital May Have Led to Carelessness, Study Says," 2007, http://www.nbcnews.com/id/22263412/ns/health-health_care/t/trail-errors-led-wrong-brain-surgeries/#.VedHytNVhBc.

17. Hemadri Makani to Success in Healthcare, September 14, 2012, http://successinhealthcare.blogspot.com/2012/10/mark-site-campaign.html.

18. Comment on operating room conversation: This conversation reportedly occurred in a hospital in India, but a version of this has played out countless times in American hospitals and the world over.

19. World Health Organization, "WHO Guidelines for Safe Surgery (First Edition)" (Geneva, Switzerland: World Health Organization, 2008).

20. R. L. Brooks, "Are You Using the Universal Protocol Yet?" *AAOS Now* 9, no. 5 (2015), http://www.aaos.org/news/bulletin/marapr07/clinical6.asp.

21. Comment regarding presurgical markings: The Universal Protocol makes accommodations for the situations in which a site marking is not anatomically or technically possible (e.g., minimal access procedures involving a lateralized organ) or when it would be undesirable to use (premature infants for whom a mark could cause a permanent tattoo), or when a patient refuses to have their body marked.

22. Martin A. Makary et al., "Operating Room Briefings and Wrong-Site Surgery," *Journal of the American College of Surgery* 204, no. 236–43 (2007).

23. Gawande, *The Checklist Manifesto*.

24. National Public Radio, "Atul Gawande's 'Checklist' for Surgery Success," *Morning Edition* (2010), http://www.npr.org/templates/story/story.php?storyId=122226184.

25. National Public Radio, "Atul Gawande's 'Checklist' for Surgery Success," 157.

26. Brooks, "Are You Using the Universal Protocol Yet?"

27. Gawande, *The Checklist Manifesto*, 160–61.

28. National Public Radio, "Atul Gawande's 'Checklist' for Surgery Success."

29. National Public Radio, "Atul Gawande's 'Checklist' for Surgery Success," 151.

30. Mary Blanco, John R. Clarke, and Denise Martindell, "Wrong Site Surgery Near Misses and Actual Occurences," *AORN Journal* 90, no. 2 (2009); John R. Clarke, "The Use of Collaboration to Implement Evidence-Based Safe Practices," *Journal of Public Health Research* 2, no. 150–53 (2013).

31. John R. Clarke, "Is Your Office Helping You Prevent Wrong Site Surgery?" *Bulletin* 99, no. 4 (2014), http://bulletin.facs.org/2014/04/is-your-office-helping-you-prevent-wrong-site-surgery/.

32. Jesse M. Pines et al., "Procedural Safety in Emergency Care: A Conceptual Model and Recommendations," *Joint Commission Journal on Quality and Patient Safety* 38, no. 11 (2012).

33. Clarke, Johnson, and Finley, "Getting Surgery Right."

CHAPTER 5

1. Sorrel King, *Josie's Story: A Mother's Inspiring Crusade to Make Medical Care Safer* (New York: Atlantic Monthly Press, 2009).

2. King, *Josie's Story*.

3. King, *Josie's Story*.

4. Maureen Maurer et al., "Guide to Patient and Family Engagement: Environmental Scan Report," in *AHRQ Publication No. 12-0042-EF* (Rockville, MD: Agency for Healthcare Research and Quality, 2012).

5. Paul L Aronson et al., "Impact of Family Presence During Pediatric Intensive Care Unit Rounds on the Family and Medical Team," *Pediarics* 124, no. 4 (2009).

6. Tom Delbanco et al., "Healthcare in a Land Called PeoplePower: Nothing About Me without Me," *Health Expectations* 4, no. 3 (2001).

7. National Patient Safety Foundation, "National Agenda for Action: Patients and Families in Patient Safety—Nothing About Me, without Me," https://c.ymcdn.com/sites/www.npsf.org/resource/collection/ABAB3CA8 -4E0A-41C5-A480-6DE8B793536C/Nothing_About_Me.pdf.

8. Wenjun Zhong et al., "Age and Sex Patterns of Drug Prescribing in a Defined American Population," Mayo Clinic Proceedings, *Mayo Clinic* 88, no. 7 (2013).

9. Medical News Today, "Record 4.02 Billion Prescriptions in the United States in 2011," *MNT* (2012), http://www.medicalnewstoday.com/ releases/250213.php.

10. Consumer Healthcare Products Association, "Statistics on OTC Use," 2015, http://www.chpa.org/marketstats.aspx.

11. J. Lazarou, B. H. Pomeranz, and P. N. Corey, "Incidence of Adverse Drug Reactions in Hospitalized Patients: A Meta-Analysis of Prospective Studies," *JAMA* 279, no. 15 (1998).

12. John Sandars and Gary Cook, *ABC of Patient Safety* (Malden, MA: Blackwell Publishing, 2007).

13. Centers for Disease Control and Prevention, "Therapeutic Drug Use," *FastStats* (2015), http://www.cdc.gov/nchs/fastats/drug-use-therapeutic.htm.

14. David C. Radley et al., "Reduction in Medication Errors in Hospitals Due to Adoption of Computerized Provider Order Entry Systems," *Journal of the American Medical Informatics Association* 20, no. 3 (2013).

15. Dianne E. Tobias and Mark Sey, "General and Psychotherapeutic Medication Use in 328 Nursing Facilities: A Year 2000 National Survey," *Consultant Pharmacist* 16, no. 1 (2001).

16. Dan Mendelson et al., "Prescription Drugs in Nursing Homes: Managing Costs and Quality in a Complex Environment," in *NHPF Issue Brief* (National Health Policy Forum, 2002).

17. T. J. Moore, M. R. Cohen, and C. D. Furberg, "Serious Adverse Drug Events Reported to the Food and Drug Administration, 1998–2005," *Archives of Internal Medicine* 167, no. 16 (2007).

18. Jill Van Den Bos et al., "The $17.1 Billion Problem: The Annual Cost of Measurable Medical Errors," *Health Affairs* 30, no. 4 (2011).

19. Institute of Medicine, "Preventing Medication Errors" (Washington, DC: National Academy Press, 2006).

20. Philip Aspden et al., *Preventing Medication Errors* (Washington, DC: National Academies Press, 2007).

21. J. D. Birkmeyer and J. B. Dimick, "Leapfrog Safety Standards: Potential Benefits of Universal Adoption," in *Fact Sheet: Computerized Physician Order Entry* (The Leapfrog Group, 2014).

22. D. W. Bates et al., "Effect of Computerized Physician Order Entry and a Team Intervention on Prevention of Serious Medication Errors," *Journal of the American Medical Association* 280 (1998).

23. Daniel R. Levinson, "Adverse Events in Skilled Nursing Facilities: National Incidence among Medicare Beneficiaries" (Washington, DC: Department of Health and Human Services, 2014).

24. D. W. Bates et al., "The Costs of Adverse Drug Events in Hospitalized Patients," *JAMA* 277, no. 4 (1997).

25. Jonathon Halbesleben et al., "Rework and Workarounds in Nurse Medication Administration Process: Implications for Work Processes and Patient Safety," *Health Care Management Review* 35, no. 2 (2010): 125.

26. L. L. Leape et al., "Systems Analysis of Adverse Drug Events," *JAMA* 274, no. 1 (1995).

27. Robert K. Michaels et al., "Achieving the National Quality Forum's 'Never Events': Prevention of Wrong Site, Wrong Procedure, and Wrong Patient Operations," *Annals of Surgery* 245, no. 4 (2007).

28. Matthew Grissinger, "The Five Rights: A Destination without a Map," *Pharmacy and Therapeutics* 35, no. 10 (2010).

29. T. A. Brennan et al., "Incidence of Adverse Events and Negligence in Hospitalized Patients: Results from the Harvard Medical Practice Study," *New England Journal of Medicine* 324 (1991).

30. The Leapfrog Group, "Fact Sheet: Computerized Physician Order Entry," http://www.leapfroggroup.org/media/file/FactSheet_CPOE.pdf.

31. Leah Binder and William H. Finck, "Results of the 2013 Leapfrog Hospital Survey: Executive Summary" (2015), http://www.leapfroggroup.org/sites/default/files/Files/2013LeapfrogHospitalSurveyResultsReport.pdf.

32. Castlight Health, "Results of the 2014 Leapfrog Hospital Survey: Computerized Physician Order Entry," 2015.

33. The Leapfrog Group, "Factsheet: Bar Code Medication Administration," http://www.leapfroggroup.org/sites/default/files/Files/BCMA_Fact Sheet.pdf.

34. Larry Mercer, Philip Felt, and Noell R. Snider, "Getting the Most Out of Your Epic EMR Training Program," *White Paper* (2012), http://divurgent.com/wp-content/uploads/pdf/EpicEMRTrainingProgram.pdf.

35. Del Beccaro, H. E. Jeffries, M. A. Eisenberg, and E. D. Harry, "Computerized Provider Order Entry Implementation: No Association with Increased Morality Rates in an Intensive Care Unit," *Pediatrics* 118, no. 1 (2006).

36. CBS, "Hospital Agrees to Pay $8.25M in Baby's Death from Overdose," *CBS Chicago* (2012), http://chicago.cbslocal.com/2012/04/05/babys-death-yields-record-settlement-of-more-than-8m/.

37. D. Dowell, T. M. Haegerich, and R. Chou, "CDC Guideline for Prescribing Opioids for Chronic Pain—United States, 2016," *JAMA* 315, no. 15 (2016).

38. CBS, "Hospital Agrees to Pay $8.25M in Baby's Death from Overdose."

39. Bibb Latane and Judith Rodin, "A Lady in Distress: Inhibiting Effects of Friends and Strangers on Bystander Intervention," *Journal of Experimental Social Psychology* 5 (1969).

40. Megan McArdle, *The Up Side of Down: Why Failing Well Is the Key to Success* (New York: Penquin Books, 2015).

41. Department of Education, "Human Performance Improvement Handbook" (Washington, DC: U.S. Depatment of Energy, 2009).

42. Whatis.com, "Workaround," http://whatis.techtarget.com/definition/workaround.

43. Leslie Kirle, "Errors in Transcribing and Administering Medications," *Safety First Alert* (2001), http://www.macoalition.org/documents/SafetyFirst3.pdf.

44. "Workarounds to Barcode Medication Administration Systems: Their Occurrences, Causes, and Threats to Patient Safety," *Journal of the American Medical Informatics Association* 15, no. 4 (2008).

45. Aaron S. Kesselheim et al., "Clinical Decision Support Systems Could Be Modified to Reduce 'Alert Fatigue' While Still Minimizing the Risk of Litigation," *Health Affairs* 30, no. 12 (2011).

46. Heleen van der Sijs et al., "Overriding of Drug Safety Alerts in Computerized Physician Order Entry," *Journal of the American Medical Informatics Association: JAMIA* 13, no. 2 (2006).

47. Institute for Safe Medication Practices, "The Five Rights: A Destination without a Map," https://www.ismp.org/newsletters/acutecare/articles/20070125.asp.

48. Grissinger, "The Five Rights: A Destination without a Map."

49. Institute for Safe Medication Practices, "The Five Rights."

50. World Health Organization, "Patient Identification," *Patient Safety Solutions* 1, Solution 2 (2007), http://www.who.int/patientsafety/solutions/patientsafety/PS-Solution2.pdf.

51. Maurer et al., "Guide to Patient and Family Engagement."

52. National Patient Safety Agency, "Wristbands for Hospital Inpatients Improves Safety," http://www.nrls.npsa.nhs.uk/EasySiteWeb/getresource.axd?AssetID=60032.

53. Institute for Safe Medication Practices, "Independent Double-Checks: Undervalued and Misused," Institute for Safe Medication Practices, https://www.ismp.org/newsletters/acutecare/showarticle.aspx?id=51.

54. PR Newswire, "Boston Medical Center Teams up with Rhode Island Hospital, CVS Health to Address Use of Pharmacy-Based Naloxone to Combat Opioid Addiction and Overdoses," news release, 2015, http://www.prnewswire.com/news-releases/boston-medical-center-teams-up-with-rhode-island-hospital-cvs-health-to-address-use-of-pharmacy-based-naloxone-to-combat-opioid-addiction-and-overdoses-300124914.html.

55. Carolyn Weems, "Fighting Heroin in Virginia Beach," *Virginian-Pilot*, November 20, 2015.

56. Margaret Kavanagh, "Virginia Beach School Board Member Shares Painful Memories of Daughter's Overdose," WTKR, July 8, 2015.

57. Sam Quinones, *Dreamland: The True Tale of America's Opiate Epidemic* (Dexter, MI: Bloomsbury Press, 2015).

58. Substance Abuse and Mental Health Service Administration, "Results from the 2013 National Survey on Drug Use and Health: Summary of National Findings," ed. Substance Abuse and Mental Health Service Administration (Rockville, MD, 2014).

59. Centers for Disease Control and Prevention, "New Research Reveals the Trends and Risk Factors Behind America's Growing Heroin Epidemic," news release, July 7, 2015, 2015, http://www.cdc.gov/media/releases/2015/p0707-heroin-epidemic.html.

60. Gretchen LeFever Watson, Andrea Powell Arcona, and David O. Antonuccio, "The ADHD Drug Abuse Crisis on American College Campuses," *Ethical Human Psychology and Psychiatry* 17, no. 1 (2015); Gretchen LeFever Watson et al., "Shooting the Messenger: The Case of ADHD," *Journal of Contemporary Psychotherapy* 44, no. 1 (2014); Gretchen LeFever Watson, "The Deadly Dangers of ADHD Drugs," *Virginian-Pilot*, October 2, 2016.

61. United Nations Office on Drugs and Crime, "Word Drug Report 2012," http://www.unodc.org/unodc/en/data-and-analysis/WDR-2012.html.

62. Alexandra Robbins, *The Nurses: A Year of Secrets, Drama, and Miracles with the Heroes of the Hospital* (New York: Workman Publishing Company, Inc., 2015).

63. Patricia Borns, "Investigation: Addicted Nurses Steal Patients' Drugs: In Virginia, a Broken System of Employers and State Programs Allow It to Continue," *Investigation: Addicted Nurses* (2016), http://www.newsleader.com/topic/997446b5-cea1-4493-b989-548be165cc47/addicted-nurses/.

64. Donna Tartt, *The Goldfinch* (New York: Little, Brown and Company, 2013).

65. Mark Herring, "An Epidemic of Opioid Death," *Virginian-Pilot*, September 21, 2016.

66. Kavanagh, "Virginia Beach School Board Member Shares Painful Memories of Daughter's Overdose."

67. Borns, "Investigation: Addicted Nurses Steal Patients' Drugs."

68. Centers for Disease Control and Prevention, "Therapeutic Drug Use."

69. Dowell, Haegerich, and Chou, "CDC Guideline for Prescribing Opioids for Chronic Pain—United States, 2016."

CHAPTER 6

1. National Patient Safety Foundation, "Safety Is Personal: Partnering with Patients and Families for the Safest Care" (Boston, MA: National Patient Safety Foundation, 2014).

2. Tejal K. Gandhi and Gregg S. Meyer, "United for Patient Safety: National Patient Safety Foundation Report 2014–2015" (Boston, MA: National Patient Safety Foundation, 2016).

3. Vikki Entwistle, Michelle M. Mello, and Troyen A. Brennan, "Advising Patients About Patient Safety: Current Initiatives Risk Shifting Responsibility," *Journal on Quality and Patient Safety* 31, no. 9 (2005).

4. Vikki Entwistle, "Nursing Shortages and Patient Safety Problems in Hospital Care: Is Clinical Monitoring by Families Part of the Solution?" *Health Expectations* 7 (2004).

5. Joint Commission on Accreditation of Healthcare Organizations, "Speak Up: Help Prevent Errors in Your Care," in *JCAHCO*, ed. Joint Commission on Accreditation of Health Care Organizations (2003).

6. G. Van Kanegan and M. Boyette, *How to Survive Your Hospital Stay: The Complete Guide to Getting the Care You Need—and Avoiding Problems You Don't* (New York: Fireside, 2003).

7. Richard Pascale, Jerry Sternin, and Monique Sternin, *The Power of Positive Deviance: How Unlikely Innovators Solve the World's Toughest Problems* (Boston, MA: Harvard Business Press, 2010).

8. Arvind Singhal and Karen Greiner, "Do What You Can with What You Have, Where You Are Now: A Quest to Eliminate MRSA at the VA Pittsburgh Healthcare System," *Deeper Learning* 1, no. 4 (2007).

9. Singhal and Greiner, "Do What You Can with What You Have," 6.

10. Pascale, Sternin, and Sternin, *The Power of Positive Deviance*; Singhal and Greiner, "Do What You Can with What You Have."

11. Singhal and Greiner, "Do What You Can with What You Have," 12.

12. Comment on positive deviance work at the VA: The VA Pittsburgh Healthcare System's website includes updates on its positive deviance work, but such postings ended in 2008. By the time the manuscript for this book was submitted to the publisher, nobody had responded to requests for an update on the initiative or its diffusion to other facilities.

13. Pascale, Sternin, and Sternin, *The Power of Positive Deviance*.

14. Noreen M. Clark et al., "Community Coalitions to Control Chronic Disease: Allies against Asthma as a Model and Case Study," *Health Promotion Practice* 7, no. 2 (Supplement) (2006); G. B. LeFever, F. D. Butterfoss, and N. Vislocky, "High Prevalence of Attention Deficit Hyperactivity Disorder: Catalyst for Development of a School Health Coalition," *Family and Community Health* 22, no. 1 (1999); K. M. Mack, C. S. Kelly, and A. L. Morrow, "Head Start: A Setting for Asthma Outreach and Prevention," *Community Health* 22, no. 1.

15. J. A. Alexander et al., "Sustainability of Collaborative Capacity in Community Health Partnerships," *Medical Research and Review* 60, no. 4 (2003); P. G. Foster-Fishman et al., "Building Collaborative Capacity in Community Coalitions: A Review and Integrative Framework," *American Journal of Community Psychology* 29, no. 2241–261 (2001).

16. Clark et al., "Community Coalitions to Control Chronic Disease."

17. Alexander et al., "Sustainability of Collaborative Capacity in Community Health Partnerships"; Foster-Fishman et al., "Building Collaborative Capacity in Community Coalitions."

18. Comment on steps for building a community coalition: The steps in the table at the end of this chapter represent an adaptation of material that was posted on the Illinois attorney general's website.

19. G. B. LeFever, A. P. Arcona, and D. O. Antonuccio, "ADHD among American Schoolchildren: Evidence of Overdiagnosis and Overuse of Medication," *Scientific Review of Mental Health Practice* 2, no. 1 (2003); LeFever, Butterfoss, and Vislocky, "High Prevalence of Attention Deficit Hyperactivity Disorder"; G. B. LeFever et al., "Understanding ADHD Issues in a Community with a High ADHD Prevalence Rate: Parent, Teacher, and Provider Prespectives," in *128th Annual Meeting of the American Public Health Association* (Boston, MA, 2000); G. B. LeFever et al., "Parental Perceptions of Adverse Educational Outcomes among Children Diagnosed with ADHD: A Call for Improved School/Provider Collaboration," *Psychology in the Schools* 39, no. 1 (2002).

20. G. B. LeFever, "Issue Brief: Increased Use of Psychiatric Drugs in American Schools" (Arlington, VA: The Lexington Institute, 2002); LeFever,

Arcona, and Antonuccio, "ADHD among American Schoolchildren"; G. B. LeFever, K. V. Dawson, and A. L. Morrow, "The Extent of Drug Therapy for Attention-Deficit/Hyperactivity Disorder among Children in Public Schools," *American Journal of Public Health* 89, no. 9 (1999).

21. G. B. LeFever, K. Allen, and E. A. Plasden, "Piloting a School-Wide Behavioral Intervention Study," in *132nd Annual Meeting of the American Public Health Association* (Washington, DC, 2004).

22. Gretchen LeFever Watson et al., "Shooting the Messenger: The Case of ADHD," *Journal of Contemporary Psychotherapy* 44, no. 1 (2014).

23. Gretchen LeFever Watson, Andrea Powell Arcona, and David O. Antonuccio, "The ADHD Drug Abuse Crisis on American College Campuses," *Ethical Human Psychology and Psychiatry* 17, no. 1 (2015).

24. S. N. Visser et al., "Trends in the Parent-Report of Health Care Provider-Diagnosed and Medicated Attention-Deficit/Hyperactivity Disorder: United States, 2003–2011," *Journal of the American Academy of Child & Adolescent Psychiatry* (2013).

25. A. Schwarz, "The Selling of Attention Deficit Disorder," *New York Times*, December 14, 2013; Watson, Arcona, and Antonuccio, "The ADHD Drug Abuse Crisis on American College Campuses."

26. G. L. Watson and A. P. Arcona, "8 Ways to Respond to Student ADHD Drug Abuse," *Campus Safety*, 2014; "ADHD Drug Abuse Epidemic Prompts New School Rules," *Campus Safety*, May 3, 2014; Watson, Arcona, and Antonuccio, "The ADHD Drug Abuse Crises on American College Campuses."

27. Watson, Arcona, and Antonuccio, "The ADHD Drug Abuse Crises on American College Campuses."

28. Martin A. Makary and Michael Daniel, "Medical Error—the Third Leading Cause of Death in the US," *BMJ* 353 (2016).

29. National Patient Safety Foundation, http://www.npsf.org/?page=aboutus.

30. The group did not meet all community coalition criteria in that membership was not open to the public; it was based on an application process.

31. G. B. LeFever, "Chasing Zero Events of Harm: An Urgent Call to Expand Safety Culture Work and Patient Engagement," *Nursing and Patient Care* (February 2010), http://www.yoursls.com/ConnectingHospitals -Communities.pdf.

32. James L Reinertsen, Michael D. Bisgnano, and Maureen Pugh, "Seven Leadership Leverage Points for Organizational-Level Improvement in Health Care" (Cambridge, MA: Institute for Healthcare Improvement, 2008), 17.

33. National Patient Safety Foundation, "Safety Is Personal: Partnering with Patients and Families for the Safest Care," xiii.

CHAPTER 7

1. Arthur Conan Doyle, *The Complete Sherlock Holmes* (New York: Bantam Classics, 1986).

2. George David Smith and Frederick Dalzell, *Wisdom from the Robber Barons: Enduring Lessons from Rockefeller, Morgan, and the First Industrialists* (New York: Basic Books, 2000).

3. Alexandra Robbins, *The Nurses: A Year of Secrets, Drama, and Miracles with the Heroes of the Hospital* (New York: Workman Publishing Company, Inc., 2015).

4. Melanie E deWit et al., "Supporting Second Victims of Patient Safety Events: Shouldn't These Communications Be Covered by Legal Privilege?" *Journal of Law, Medicine, and Ethics* (Winter 2013); Stephen Pratt et al., "How to Develop a Second Victim Support Program: A Toolkit for Health Care Organizations," *Joint Commission Journal on Quality and Patient Safety* 38, no. 5 (2012); Susan D. Scott, "The 'Second Victim' Phenomenon: A Harsh Reality of Health Care Professions," *Perpectives on Safety* (May 2011), https://psnet.ahrq.gov/perspectives/perspective/102.

5. Carolyn M Clancy, "Alleviating 'Secondary Victim' Syndrome: How We Should Handle Patient Harm?" *Journal of Nursing Care Quality* 27, no. 1 (2012); Scott, "The 'Second Victim' Phenomenon"; Albert W. Wu et al., "Disclosure of Adverse Events in the United States and Canada: An Update, and a Proposed Framework for Improvement," *Journal of Public Health Research* 2, no. 3 (2013).

6. Albert W. Wu, "Medical Error: The Second Victim: The Doctor Who Makes the Mistake Needs Help Too," *BMJ: British Medical Journal* 320, no. 7237 (2000): 726–27.

7. Clancy, "Alleviating 'Secondary Victim' Syndrome."

8. Pratt et al., "How to Develop a Second Victim Support Program."

9. Jane Garbutt et al., "Reporting and Disclosing Medical Errors: Pediatricians' Attitudes and Behaviors," *Archives of Pediatric and Adolescent Medicine* 16, no. 2 (2007).

10. Robbins, *The Nurses*.

11. deWit et al., "Supporting Second Victims of Patient Safety Events."

12. Samuel Gorovitz and Alasdair MacIntyre, "Toward a Theory of Medical Fallibility," *Hastings Center Report* (December 1975).

13. Elizabeth A. McGlynn et al., "The Quality of Health Care Delivered to Adults in the United States," *New England Journal of Medicine* 348, no. 26 (2003).

14. Mark Ware and Michael Mabe, "The STM Report: An Overview of Scientific and Scholarly Publishing," in *The STM Report* (Netherlands, 2012).

15. John P. A. Ioannidis, "Why Most Published Research Findings Are False," *PLoS Medicine* 2, no. 8 (2007).

16. Shannon Brownlee, *Overtreated: Why Too Much Medicine Is Making Us Sicker and Poorer* (New York: Bloomsbury, 2008); Sandeep Jauhar, *Doctored: The Disillusionment of an American Physician* (New York: Farrar, Straus, and Giroux, 2014).

17. Gorovitz and MacIntyre, "Toward a Theory of Medical Fallibility," 13.

18. James Lyons-Weiler, in *Cures vs. Profits: Successes in Translational Research* (London: World Scientific, 2016).

19. D. H. Novack et al., "Changes in Physicians' Attitudes toward Telling the Cancer Patient," *JAMA* 241, no. 9 (1979).

20. Norman Hamilton, "Suicide of Nurse after Tragic Event," *Seattle Times*, April 22, 2011.

21. Rosemary Gibson and Janardan Prasad Singh, *Wall of Silence: The Untold Story of the Medical Mistakes That Kill and Injury Millions of Americans* (Washington, DC: LifeLine Press, 2003), 104–5.

22. Malcolm Gladwell, *Outliers: The Story of Success.* New York: Little, Brown and Company, 2008.

23. A. Schwarz, "Drowned in a Stream of Prescriptions," *New York Times*, February 2, 2013.

24. Elizabeth Simpson, "Va. Beach Psychiatrist's License to Be Suspended," *Virginian-Pilot*, October 28, 2014.

25. Megan McArdle, *The Up Side of Down: Why Failing Well Is the Key to Success* (New York: Penquin Books, 2015), 80.

26. McArdle, *The Up Side of Down*, 80.

27. McArdle, *The Up Side of Down*, 81.

28. McArdle, *The Up Side of Down*, 82.

29. Linda H Aiken et al., "Hospital Nurse Staffing and Patient Mortality, Nurse Burnout, and Job Dissatisfaction," *Journal of the American Medical Association* 288, no. 16 (2002).

30. K. Frith et al., "Nurse Staffing Is an Important Strategy to Prevent Medication Errors in Community Hospitals," *Nursing Economics* 30, no. 5 (2012).

31. T. Lewis-Voepel et al., "Nursing Surveillance Moderates the Relationship between Staffing Levels and Pediatric Postoperative Serious Adverse Events: A Nested-Case Control Study," *International Journal of Nursing Studies* 50, no. 7 (2012).

32. Institute for Safe Medication Practices, "Since When Is It a Crime to Be Human?" news release, 2006, http://www.ismp.org/pressroom/viewpoints/julie.asp.

33. T. Christine Kovner et al., "What Does Nurse Turnover Rate Mean and What Is the Rate?" *Policy, Politics, & Nursing Practice* 15, no. 3–4 (2014).

34. C. Kane, "Policy Research Perspectives—Medical Liability Claim Frequency: A 2007–2008 Snapshot of Physicians" (Chicago: American Medical Association, 2010).

35. Anupam B. Jena et al., "Malpractice Risk According to Physician Specialty," *New England Journal of Medicine* 365, no. 629–36 (2011).

36. Stephanie P. Fein et al., "The Many Faces of Error Disclosure: A Common Set of Elements and a Definition," *Journal of General Internal Medicine* 22, no. 6 (2007): 760.

37. P. J. Pronovost and E. Vohr, *Safe Patients, Smart Hospitals: How One Doctor's Checklist Can Help Us Change Health Care from the Inside Out* (New York: Penquin Group, 2010).

38. Wu et al., "Disclosure of Adverse Events in the United States and Canada."

39. Ann Hendrich et al., "Ascension Health's Demonstration of Full Disclosure Protocol for Unexpected Events During Labor and Delivery Shows Promise," *Health Affairs* 33, no. 1 (2014).

40. T. H. Gallagher et al., "US and Canadian Physicians's Attitudes and Experiences Regarding Disclosing Errors to Patients," *Archives of Internal Medicine* 166, no. 15 (2006).

41. Wu et al., "Disclosure of Adverse Events in the United States and Canada."

42. Fein et al., "The Many Faces of Error Disclosure."

43. Joshua M. Liao, Eric J. Thomas, and Sigall K. Bell, "Speaking up About the Dangers of the Hidden Curriculum," *Health Affairs* 33, no. 1 (2014): 169.

44. Gibson and Singh, *Wall of Silence.*

45. Gibson and Singh, *Wall of Silence*, 20.

46. Gibson and Singh, *Wall of Silence*, 186.

47. American Association of Colleges of Nursing, "Nursing Fact Sheet," American Association of Colleges of Nursing, http://www.aacn.nche.edu/media-relations/fact-sheets/nursing-fact-sheet.

48. Sarah E. Shannon et al., "Disclosing Errors to Patients: Perspectives of Registered Nurses," *The Joint Commission Journal on Quality and Patient Safety* 35, no. 1 (2009).

49. Deanna L. Reising and Patricia N. Allen, "Protecting Yourself from Malpractice Claims," *American Nurse Today* (February 2007).

50. Wu et al., "Disclosure of Adverse Events in the United States and Canada."

51. Sorrel King, *Josie's Story: A Mother's Inspiring Crusade to Make Medical Care Safer* (New York: Atlantic Monthly Press, 2009); Pronovost and Vohr, *Safe Patients, Smart Hospitals*.

52. G. B. Hickson et al., "Factors That Prompted Families to File Medical Malpractice Claims Following Perinatal Injuries," *Journal of the American Medical Association* 267 (1992).

53. Albert W. Wu, *Being Open with Patients and Families About Adverse Events*, podcast audio, Medical Center Hour Being Open with Patients and Families, 2010, https://www.youtube.com/watch?v=DkYm8HFq_Vk.

54. N. Varjavand, S. Nair, and E. Gracely, "A Call to Address the Curricular Provision of Emotional Support in the Event of Medical Errors and Adverse Events," *Medical Education* 46 (2012).

55. Michelle M. Mello et al., "Communication-and-Resolution Programs: The Challenges and Lessons Learned from Six Early Adopters," *Health Affairs* 33, no. 1 (2014); Michelle M. Mello et al., "Implementing Hospital-Based Communication-and-Resolution Programs: Lessons Learned in New York City."

56. Ann Hendrich et al., "Ascension Health's Demonstration of Full Disclosure Protocol for Unexpected Events During Labor and Delivery Shows Promise"; Allen Kachalia et al., "Liability Claims and Costs before and after Implementation of a Medical Error Disclosure Program," *Annals of Internal Medicine* 153, no. 4 (2010); Steve S. Kraman and Ginny Hamm, "Risk Management: Extreme Honesty May Be the Best Policy," 131, no. 12 (1999); Pronovost and Vohr, *Safe Patients, Smart Hospitals*.

57. In addition to modeling how to translate hospital policy into action, the Ascension story can serve as a blueprint of how a community coalition might implement changes that it prioritizes.

58. Hendrich et al., "Ascension Health's Demonstration of Full Disclosure Protocol for Unexpected Events During Labor and Delivery Shows Promise."

59. Wu et al., "Disclosure of Adverse Events in the United States and Canada."

60. Comment on including patients in patient safety investigations: All disclosure programs that are currently in operation may not explicitly invite patients to participate in the investigation; however, there is growing support for doing so because patients have the potential to offer unique insights for improvement and the process aids in their healing process.

61. Jason M. Etchegaray et al., "Structuring Patient and Family Involvement in Medical Error Event Disclosure and Analysis," *Health Affairs* 33, no. 1 (2014).

62. Etchegaray et al., "Structuring Patient and Family Involvement in Medical Error Event Disclosure and Analysis."

63. Etchegaray et al., "Structuring Patient and Family Involvement in Medical Error Event Disclosure and Analysis."

64. deWit et al., "Supporting Second Victims of Patient Safety Events."

65. Kachalia et al., "Liability Claims and Costs before and after Implementation of a Medical Error Disclosure Program."

66. John K Iglehart, "Improved Safety, Eliminating Errors Top Policy Agenda," *Health Affairs* 33, no. 1 (2014).

67. Allen Kachalia et al., "Greatest Impact of Safe Harbor Rule May Be to Improve Patient Safety, Not Reduce Liability Claims Paid by Physicians."

68. David M. Studdert et al., "Claims, Errors, and Compensation Payments in Medical Malpractice Litigation," *New England Journal of Medicine* 354, no. 19 (2006).

69. David M. Studdert, Michelle M. Mello, and Troyen A. Brennan, "Medical Malpractice," *New England Journal of Medicine* 350, no. 3 (2004).

70. deWit et al., "Supporting Second Victims of Patient Safety Events."

71. Gorovitz and MacIntyre, "Toward a Theory of Medical Fallibility."

Bibliography

Aiken, Linda H., Sean P. Clarke, Douglas M. Sloane, Julie Sochalski, and Jeffrey H Silber. "Hospital Nurse Staffing and Patient Mortality, Nurse Burnout, and Job Dissatisfaction." *Journal of the American Medical Association* 288, no. 16 (2002): 1987–93.

Alexander, J. A., B. J. Weiner, M. E. Metzger, S. M. Shortell, G. J. Bazzoli, and R. Hasnain-Wynia. "Sustainability of Collaborative Capacity in Community Health Partnerships." *Medical Care Research and Review* 60, no. 4 (2003): 130S–60S.

American Association of Colleges of Nursing. "Nursing Fact Sheet." American Association of Colleges of Nursing. http://www.aacn.nche.edu/media-relations/fact-sheets/nursing-fact-sheet.

Andel, C., S. L. Davidow, M. Hollander, and D. A. Moreno. "The Economics of Health Care Quality and Medical Errors." *Journal of Health Care Finance* 39, no. 1 (Fall 2012): 39–50.

Aronson, Paul L., Jennifer Yau, Mark A. Helfaer, and Wynne Morrison. "Impact of Family Presence during Pediatric Intensive Care Unit Rounds on the Family and Medical Team." *Pediatrics* 124, no. 4 (2009): 1119–25.

Aspden, Philip, Julie A. Wolcott, J. Lyle Bootman, and Linda R. Cronewett. *Preventing Medication Errors*. Washington, DC: National Academies Press, 2007.

Associated Press. "Trail of Errors Led to 3 Wrong Brain Surgeries." December 14, 2007. http://www.nbcnews.com/id/22263412/ns/health-health_care/t/trail-errors-led-wrong-brain-surgeries/#.WBUSquErJTY.

———. "Trail of Errors Led to 3 Wrong Brain Surgeries: Surgeons' Ego at R.I. Hospital May Have Led to Carelessness, Study Says." December 14, 2007. http://www.nbcnews.com/id/22263412/ns/health-health_care/t/trail-errors-led-wrong-brain-surgeries/#.VedHytNVhBc.

Badjie, Ismaila D. "Presentation to Center for Medication Safety Advancement: Impact of Technology on Medication Safety." Purdue University, 2012.

Bates, D. W., L. L. Leape, D. J. Cullen, N. Laird, L. A. Petersen, J. M. Teich, E. Burdick et al. "Effect of Computerized Physician Order Entry and a Team Intervention on Prevention of Serious Medication Errors." *Journal of the American Medical Association* 280 (1998): 1311–6.

Bates, D. W., N. Spell, D. J. Cullen et al. "The Costs of Adverse Drug Events in Hospitalized Patients." *JAMA* 277, no. 4 (1997): 307–11.

Beccaro, Mark A. Del, Howard E. Jeffries, Matthew E. Eisenberg, and E. D. Harry. "Computerized Provider Order Entry Implementation: No Association with Increased Mortality Rates in an Intensive Care Unit." *Pediatrics* 118, no. 1 (2006): 290–95.

Berwick, Donald M. "What 'Patient-Centered' Should Mean: Confessions of an Extremist." *Health Affairs* 28 (2009): w55–w65.

Binder, Leah. "The Leapfrog Annual Hospital Survey." Personal communication (email), 2013.

———. "Stunning News on Preventable Deaths in Hospitals." *Forbes Magazine* (2013). September 23, 2013. http://www.forbes.com/sites/leah binder/2013/09/23/stunning-news-on-preventable-deaths-in-hospitals/.

Binder, Leah, and William H. Finck. "Results of the 2013 Leapfrog Hospital Survey: Executive Summary." July 9, 2015. http://www.leapfroggroup.org/sites/default/files/Files/2013LeapfrogHospitalSurveyResultsReport.pdf.

Birkmeyer, J. D., and J. B. Dimick. "Leapfrog Safety Standards: Potential Benefits of Universal Adoption." In *Fact Sheet: Computerized Physician Order Entry*. The Leapfrog Group, 2014.

Bittle, M. J., and S. LaMarch. "Engaging the Patient as Observer to Promote Hand Hygiene Compliance in Ambulatory Care." *The Joint Commission Journal on Quality and Patient Safety* 35, no. 10 (2009): 519–25.

Blanco, Mary, John R. Clarke, and Denise Martindell. "Wrong Site Surgery Near Misses and Actual Occurrences." *AORN Journal* 90, no. 2 (2009): 215–22.

Borns, Patricia. "Investigation: Addicted Nurses Steal Patients' Drugs: In Virginia, a Broken System of Employers and State Programs Allow It to Continue." *Investigation: Addicted Nurses* (2016). http://www.newsleader.com/topic/997446b5-cea1-4493-b989-548be165cc47/addicted-nurses/.

Brennan, T. A., L. L. Leape, N. Laird et al. "Incidence of Adverse Events and Negligence in Hospitalized Patients: Results from the Harvard Medical Practice Study." *New England Journal of Medicine* 324 (1991): 370–76.

Bria, William F. "The Electronic Health Record: Is It Meaningful Yet?" *Mayo Clinic Proceedings* 86, no. 5 (2011): 373–74.

Brooks, R. L. "Are You Using the Universal Protocol Yet?" *AAOS Now* 9, no. 5 (2015). http://www.aaos.org/news/bulletin/marapr07/clinical6.asp.

Brownlee, Shannon. *Overtreated: Why Too Much Medicine Is Making Us Sicker and Poorer.* New York: Bloomsbury, 2008.

Burke, G. H., G. B. LeFever, and S. M. Sayles. "Zero Events of Harm to Patients: Building and Sustaining a System-Wide Culture of Safety at Sentara Healthcare." *Managing Infection Control* (2009): 44–50. http://www.yoursls.com/Culture-Safety-Healthcare.pdf.

Call, Josep, Juliane Brauer, Juliane Kaminski, and Michael Tomasello. "Domestic Dogs (Canis familiaris) Are Sensitive to the Attentional State of Humans." *Comparative Psychology* 117, no. 3 (2003): 257–63.

Campbell, E. G., S. Regan, R. L. Gruen, T. G. Ferris, S. R. Rao, P. D. Cleary, and D. Blumenthal. "Professionalism in Medicine: Results of a National Survey of Physicians." *Annals of Internal Medicine* 147, no. 795 (2007): 208.

Carr, D. F. "Electronic Health Records: First, Do No Harm?" *InformationWeek.* July 1, 2014. http://www.informationweek.com/healthcare/electronic-health-records/electronic-health-records-first-do-no-harm/a/d-id/1278834.

Castlight Health. "Results of the 2014 Leapfrog Hospital Survey: Computerized Physician Order Entry." 2015.

CBS. "Hospital Agrees to Pay $8.25M in Baby's Death from Overdose." *CBS Chicago.* April 5, 2012. http://chicago.cbslocal.com/2012/04/05/babys-death-yields-record-settlement-of-more-than-8m/.

Center for Advancing Health. "A New Definition of Patient Engagement: What Is Engagement and Why Is It Important?" Washington DC, 2010.

Centers for Disease Control and Prevention. "General Information About MRSA in the Community." Centers for Disease Control and Prevention.

———. "New Research Reveals the Trends and Risk Factors Behind America's Growing Heroin Epidemic." news release, July 7, 2015. http://www.cdc.gov/media/releases/2015/p0707-heroin-epidemic.html.

———. "Therapeutic Drug Use." *FastStats.* May 14, 2015. http://www.cdc.gov/nchs/fastats/drug-use-therapeutic.htm.

Charles, D., M. Gabriel, and M. F. Furukawa. "Adoption of Electronic Health Record Systems among U.S. Non-Federal Acute Care Hospitals: 2008–2013." ONC. https://www.healthit.gov/sites/default/files/oncdatabrief16.pdf.

Chassin, M. R., and J. M. Loeb. "High-Reliability Health Care: Getting There from Here." *Milbank Quarterly* 91, no. 3 (2013): 459–90.

Clancy, Carolyn M. "Alleviating 'Secondary Victim' Syndrome: How We Should Handle Patient Harm." *Journal of Nursing Care Quality* 27, no. 1 (2012): 1–5.

Clark, Noreen M., Linda Joe Doctor, Amy R. Friedman, Laurie L. Lachance, Christy R. Houle, Xin Geng, and Jeanne Ann Grisso. "Community Coalitions to Control Chronic Disease: Allies against Asthma as a Model and Case Study." *Health Promotion Practice* 7, no. 2 (Supplement) (2006): 14S–22S.

Clarke, John R. "Is Your Office Helping You Prevent Wrong Site Surgery?" *Bulletin* 99, no. 4 (2014). http://bulletin.facs.org/2014/04/is-your-office-helping-you-prevent-wrong-site-surgery/.

———. "The Use of Collaboration to Implement Evidence-Based Safe Practices." *Journal of Public Health Research* 2, no. 150–53 (2013).

Clarke, John R., Janet Johnston, and Edward D. Finley. "Getting Surgery Right." *Annals of Surgery* 246, no. 3 (2007): 395–405.

Classen, D. C., R. Resar, F. Griffin, F. Federico, T. Frankel, N. Kimmel, J. C. Whittington et al. "'Global Trigger Tool' Shows That Adverse Events in Hospitals May Be Ten Times Greater Than Previously Measured." *Health Affairs* 30, no. 58 (2011): 1–9.

Consumer Healthcare Products Association. "Statistics on OTC Use." (2015). http://www.chpa.org/marketstats.aspx.

Coulter, Angela, and Jo Ellins. "Effectiveness of Strategies for Informing, Educating, and Involving Patients." *BMJ: British Medical Journal* 335, no. 7609: 24–27.

Cummings, K. L., D. J. Anderson, and K. S. Kaye. "Hand Hygiene Noncompliance and the Cost of Hospital-Acquired Methicillin-Resistant Staphylococcus aureus Infection." *Infection Control and Hospital Epidemiology* 31, no. 4 (2010): 357–64.

Deis, J. N., K. M. Smith, M. D. Warren, P. G. Throop, G. B. Hickson, B. J. Joers, and J. K. Deshpande. "Transforming the Morbidity and Mortality Conference into an Instrument for Systemwide Improvement." In *Advances in Patient Safety: New Directions and Alternative Approaches*, edited by K. Henriksen, J. B. Battles, and M. A. Keyes. Rockville, MD: Agency for Healthcare Research and Quality, 2008.

Delbanco, Tom, Donald M. Berwick, Jo Ivey Boufford, S. Edgman-Levitan, Günter Ollenschläger, Diane Plamping, and Richard G. Rockefeller. "Healthcare in a Land Called PeoplePower: Nothing About Me without Me." *Health Expectations* 4, no. 3 (2001): 144–50.

Denham Charles R., P. Angood, D. Berwick et al. "The Chasing Zero Department: Making Idealized Design a Reality." *Journal of Patient Safety* 5, no. 210–215 (2009a).

Denham, Charles R., Peter Angood, Don Berwick, Leah Binder, Carolyn M. Clancy, Janet M. Corrigan, and David Hunt. "Chasing Zero: Can Reality Meet the Rhetoric?" *Journal of Patient Safety* 5, no. 4 (2009b): 216–22.

———. "The Vital Link Department: Making Idealized Design a Reality." *Journal of Patient Safety* 5, no. 4 (2009): 216–22.

Department of Education. "Human Performance Improvement Handbook." Washington, DC: U.S. Depatment of Energy, 2009.

deWit, Melanie E., Clifford M. Marks, Jeffrey P. Natterman, and Albert W. Wu. "Supporting Second Victims of Patient Safety Events: Shouldn't These Communications Be Covered by Legal Privilege?" *Journal of Law, Medicine, and Ethics* (Winter 2013): 2–8.

Doak, Cecelia Conrath, Leonard G. Doak, and Jane H. Root. "The Literacy Problem." In *Teaching Patients with Low Literacy Skills*, 1–9. Philadelphia: J. B. Lippincott Co., 1996.

Dowell, D., T. M. Haegerich, and R. Chou. "CDC Guideline for Prescribing Opioids for Chronic Pain—United States, 2016." *JAMA* 315, no. 15 (2016): 1624–45.

Doyle, Arthur Conan. *The Complete Sherlock Holmes*. New York: Bantam Classics, 1986.

Duhigg, C. *The Power of Habit: Why We Do What We Do in Life and Business*. New York: Random House, 2014.

Duncan, Christopher Paul, and Carol Dealey. "Patients' Feelings About Hand Washing, MRSA Status and Patient Information." *British Journal of Nursing* 16, no. 1 (2007): 34–38.

Entwistle, Vikki. "Nursing Shortages and Patient Safety Problems in the Hospital Care: Is Clinical Monitoring by Families Part of the Solution?" *Health Expectations* 7 (2004): 1–5.

Entwistle, Vikki, Michelle M. Mello, and Troyen A. Brennan. "Advising Patients About Patient Safety: Current Initiatives Risk Shifting Responsibility." *Journal on Quality and Patient Safety* 31, no. 9 (2005): 483–94.

Epstein, Randi Hutter. *Get Me Out: A History of Childbirth from the Garden of Eden to the Sperm Bank*. New York: W. W. Norton and Company, 2010.

Etchegaray, Jason M., Madelene J. Ottosen, Landrus Burress, William M. Sage, Sigall K. Bell, Thomas H. Gallagher, and Eric J. Thomas. "Structuring Patient and Family Involvement in Medical Error Event Disclosure and Analysis." *Health Affairs* 33, no. 1 (2014): 46–52.

Fawcett, S. B., A. Paine-Andrews, V. T. Francisco, J. A. Schultz, K. P. Richter, R. K. Lewis, E. L. Williams et al. "Using Empowerment Theory in Collaborative Partnership for Community Health and Development." *American Journal of Community Psychology* 23, no. 5 (1995): 677–97.

Fein, Stephanie P., Lee H. Hilborne, Eugene M. Spiritus, Gregory B. Seymann, Craig R. Keenan, Kaveh G. Shojania, Marjorie Kagawa-Singer, and

Neil S. Wenger. "The Many Faces of Error Disclosure: A Common Set of Elements and a Definition." *Journal of General Internal Medicine* 22, no. 6 (2007): 755–61.

Foster-Fishman, P. G., S. L. Berkowitz, D. W. Lounsbury, S. Jacobson, and N. A. Allen. "Building Collaborative Capacity in Community Coalitions: A Review and Integrative Framework." *American Journal of Community Psychology* 29, no. 2241–261 (2001).

Frith, K., E. Anderson, F. Tseng, and E. Fong. "Nurse Staffing Is an Important Strategy to Prevent Medication Errors in Community Hospitals." *Nursing Economics* 30, no. 5 (2012): 288–94.

Gallagher, T. H., A. D. Waterman, J. M. Garbutt et al. "US and Canadian Physicians' Attitudes and Experiences Regarding Disclosing Errors to Patients." *Archives of Internal Medicine* 166, no. 15 (2006): 1605–11.

Gandhi, Tejal K., and Gregg S. Meyer. "United for Patient Safety: National Patient Safety Foundation Report 2014–2015." Boston, MA: National Patient Safety Foundation, 2016.

Garbutt, Jane, D. R. Brownstein, E. J. Klein, Amy D. Waterman, M. J. Krauss, E. K. Marcuse, Erik Hazel et al. "Reporting and Disclosing Medical Errors: Pediatricians' Attitudes and Behaviors." *Archives of Pediatric and Adolescent Medicine* 16, no. 2 (2007): 179–85.

Gardner, A. "Surgery Mix-Ups Surprisingly Common." October 18, 2010. http://www.cnn.com/2010/HEALTH/10/18/health.surgery.mixups.common/.

Gawande, A. *The Checklist Manifesto: How to Get Things Right*. New York: Metropolitan Books, 2009.

Gibson, Rosemary, and Janardan Prasad Singh. *Wall of Silence: The Untold Story of the Medical Mistakes That Kill and Injure Millions of Americans*. Washington, DC: LifeLine Press, 2003.

Gladwell, Malcolm. *Outliers: The Story of Success*. New York: Little, Brown and Company, 2008.

Gorovitz, Samuel, and Alasdair MacIntyre. "Toward a Theory of Medical Fallibility." *Hastings Center Report* (December 1975): 13–23.

Grissinger, Matthew. "The Five Rights: A Destination without a Map." *Pharmacy and Therapeutics* 35, no. 10 (2010): 542.

Grol, R., D. M. Berwick, and M. Wensing. "On the Trail of Quality and Safety in Health Care." *BMJ: British Medical Journal* 336, no. 7635 (2008): 74–76.

Halbesleben, Jonathon, R. B. Grant Savage, Douglas S. Wakefield, and Bonnie J. Wakefield. "Rework and Workarounds in Nurse Medication Administration Process: Implications for Work Processes and Patient Safety." *Health Care Management Review* 35, no. 2 (2010): 124–33.

Hamilton, Norman. "Suicide of Nurse after Tragic Event." *Seattle Times*, April 22, 2011.

Hardin, Garrett. "The Tragedy of the Commons." *Science* 162, no. 13 (1968): 1243–48.

Heath, Chip, and Dan Heath. *Made to Stick: Why Some Ideas Survive and Others Die*. New York: Random House, 2007.

Hendrich, Ann, Christine Kocot McCoy, Jane Gale, Lora Sparkman, and Palmira Santos. "Ascension Health's Demonstration of Full Disclosure Protocol for Unexpected Events During Labor and Delivery Shows Promise." *Health Affairs* 33, no. 1 (2014): 39–45.

Herring, Mark. "An Epidemic of Opioid Death." *The Virginian-Pilot*, September 21, 2016.

Hibbard, Judith H., Ellen Peters, Paul Slovic, and Martin Tusler. "Can Patients Be Part of the Solution? Views on Their Role in Preventing Medical Errors." *Medical Care Research and Review* 62, no. 5 (October 1, 2005): 601–16.

Hibbard, J. H., J. Stockard, and M. Tusler. "Does Publicizing Hospital Performance Stimulate Quality Improvement Efforts?" *Health Affairs* 22, no. 2 (2003): 84–94.

Hickson, G. B., E. W. Clayton, P. B. Githens, and F. A. Sloan. "Factors That Prompted Families to File Medical Malpractice Claims Following Perinatal Injuries." *Journal of the American Medical Association* 267 (1992): 1359–63.

Iglehart, John K. "Improved Safety, Eliminating Errors Top Policy Agenda." *Health Affairs* 33, no. 1 (2014): 6.

Infection Control Today. "Hospitals Pair Germ-Killing Robots with CDC Protocols to Protect against Ebola Virus." *Infection Control Today*, October 30, 2014. http://www.infectioncontroltoday.com/news/2014/10/hospitals-pair -germkilling-robots-with-cdc-protocols-to-protect-against-ebola-virus.aspx.

Institute for Safe Medication Practices. "The Five Rights: A Destination Without a Map." https://www.ismp.org/newsletters/acutecare/articles/20070125.asp.

———. "Independent Double-Checks: Undervalued and Misused." https:// www.ismp.org/newsletters/acutecare/showarticle.aspx?id=51.

———. "Since When Is It a Crime to Be Human?" news release, 2006. http:// www.ismp.org/pressroom/viewpoints/julie.asp.

Institute of Medicine. "Patient Safety: Achieving a New Standard of Care." Washington, DC: National Academies Press, 2004.

———. "Preventing Medication Errors." Washington, DC: National Academy Press, 2006.

Ioannidis, John P. A. "Why Most Published Research Findings Are False." *PLoS Medicine* 2, no. 8 (2007): 696–701.

Jacquet, Jennifer. *Is Shame Necessary? New Uses for an Old Tool*. New York: Random House, 2015.

James, J. T. "A New, Evidence-Based Estimate of Patient Harms Associated with Hospital Care." *Journal of Patient Safety* 9, no. 3 (2013): 122–28.

Jauhar, Sandeep. *Doctored: The Disillusionment of an American Physician*. New York: Farrar, Straus, and Giroux, 2014.

Jena, Anupam B., Seth Seabury, Darius Lakdawalla, and Amitabh Chandra. "Malpractice Risk According to Physician Specialty." *New England Journal of Medicine* 365, no. 629–36 (2011).

Jewell, K., and L. McGiffert. "To Err Is Human—to Delay Is Deadly: Ten Years Later, a Million Lives Lost, Billions of Dollars Wasted." *Consumers Union: Nonprofit Publishers of Consumer Reports*, May 2009. http://safepatientpro ject.org/pdf/safepatientproject.org-to_delay_is_deadly-2009_05.pdf.

Joint Commission on Accreditation of Healthcare Organizations. "Speak Up: Help Prevent Errors in Your Care." In *JCAHCO*, edited by Joint Commission on Accreditation of Health Care Organizations, 2003.

Kachalia, Allen, Samuel R. Kaufman, Richard Boothman, Susan Anderson, Kathleen Welch, Sanjay Saint, and Mary A. M. Rogers. "Liability Claims and Costs before and after Implementation of a Medical Error Disclosure Program." *Annals of Internal Medicine* 153, no. 4 (2010): 213–22.

Kachalia, Allen, Alison Little, Melissa Isavoran, Lynn-Marie Crider, and Jeanene Smith. "Greatest Impact of Safe Harbor Rule May Be to Improve Patient Safety, Not Reduce Liability Claims Paid by Physicians." *Health Affairs* 33, no. 1 (2014): 59–66.

Kane, C. "Policy Research Perspectives—Medical Liability Claim Frequency: A 2007–2008 Snapshot of Physicians." Chicago: American Medical Association, 2010, 1–7.

Kane, J. M., M. Brannen, and E. Kern. "Impact of Patient Safety Mandates on Medical Education in the United States." *Journal of Patient Safety* 4, no. 2 (June 2008): 93–97.

Kavanagh, Margaret. "Virginia Beach School Board Member Shares Painful Memories of Daughter's Overdose." *The Virginian-Pilot*, July 8, 2015.

Kesselheim, Aaron S., Kathrin Cresswell, Shobha Phansalkar, David W. Bates, and Aziz Sheikh. "Clinical Decision Support Systems Could Be Modified to Reduced 'Alert Fatigue' While Still Minimizing the Risk of Litigation." *Health Affairs* 30, no. 12 (2011): 2310–17.

King, Sorrel. *Josie's Story: A Mother's Inspiring Crusade to Make Medical Care Safer*. New York: Atlantic Monthly Press, 2009.

Kirle, Leslie. "Errors in Transcribing and Administering Medications." *Safety First Alert*, January 2001. http://www.macoalition.org/documents/ SafetyFirst3.pdf.

Kirsch, Irwin S., Ann Jungeblut, Lynn Jenkins, and Andrew Kolstad. "Adult Literacy in America: A First Look at the Findings of the National Adult Literacy Survey." Office of Educational Research and Improvement: U.S. Department of Education, 2002.

Klevens, R. M., J. R. Edwards, C. L. Richards, T. C. Horan, R. P. Gaynes, D. A. Pollock, and D. M. Cardo. "Estimating Health Care-Associated Infections and Deaths in U.S. Hospitals, 2002." *Public Health Reports* 122 (2007): 160–66.

Kliff, Sarah. "Medical Errors in America Kill More People Than Aids or Drug Overdoses. Here's Why." *Vox*, April 22, 2015. http://www.vox .com/2015/1/29/7878731/medical-errors-statistics.

Kohn, L. T., J. M. Corrigan, and M. S. Donaldson. "To Err Is Human: Building a Safer Health System." Washington, DC: Institute of Medicine, 1999.

———. *To Err Is Human: Building a Safer Health System*. Edited by Institute of Medicine Committee on Quality Health Care in America. Washington, DC: National Academies Press, 2000.

Kopp, Carol. "Anatomy of a Mistake." *CBS News*, March 16, 2003. http:// www.cbsnews.com/news/anatomy-of-a-mistake-16-03-2003/.

Koppel, R., T. Wetterneck, J. Telles, and B. Karsh. "Workarounds to Barcode Medication Administration Systems: Their Occurrences, Causes, and Threats to Patient Safety." *Journal of the American Medical Informatics Association* 15, no. 4 (2008): 408–23.

Kovner, Christine T., Carol S. Brewer, Farida Fatehi, and Jin Jun. "What Does Nurse Turnover Rate Mean and What Is the Rate?" *Policy, Politics, & Nursing Practice* 15, no. 3–4 (2014): 64–71.

Kraft-Todd, Gordon, E. Yoeli, S. Bhanot, and D. Rand. "Promoting Cooperation in the Field." *Current Opinion in Behavioral Sciences* 3, no. 0 (6// 2015): 96–101.

Kraman, Steve S., and Ginny Hamm. "Risk Management: Extreme Honesty May Be the Best Policy." *Annals of Internal Medicine* 131, no. 12 (1999): 963–67.

Kumar, Sanjaya. *Fatal Care: Survive in the U.S. Health System*. Minneapolis, MN: IGI Press, 2008.

Latane, Bibb, and Judith Rodin. "A Lady in Distress: Inhibiting Effects of Friends and Strangers on Bystander Intervention." *Journal of Experimental Social Psychology* 5 (1969): 189–202.

Lazarou, J., B. H. Pomeranz, and P. N. Corey. "Incidence of Adverse Drug Reactions in Hospitalized Patients: A Meta-Analysis of Prospective Studies." *JAMA* 279, no. 15 (1998): 1200–05.

Leape, L. L. "Scope of Problem and History of Patient Safety." *Obstetric and Gynecological Clinics of North America* 35 (2008): 1–10.

Leape, L. L., D. W. Bates, D. J. Cullen et al. "Systems Analysis of Adverse Drug Events." *JAMA* 274, no. 1 (1995): 35–43.

Leape, L. L., and D. M. Berwick. "Five Years after *To Err Is Human*: What Have We Learned?" *JAMA* 293, no. 19 (2005): 2384–90.

Leape, L. L., A. G. Lawthers, T. A. Brennan, and W. G. Johnson. "Preventing Medical Injury." *Quarterly Review Bulletein* 19, no. 5 (1993): 144–49.

Leape, L. L., M. F. Shore, J. L. Dienstag et al. "Perspective: A Culture of Respect, Part 1: The Nature and Causes of Disrespectful Behavior by Physicians." *Academic Medicine* 87, no. 7 (2012): 845–52.

The Leapfrog Group. "Factsheet: Bar Code Medication Administration." http://www.leapfroggroup.org/sites/default/files/Files/BCMA_FactSheet.pdf.

———. "Fact Sheet: Computerized Physician Order Entry." http://www.leapfroggroup.org/sites/default/files/Files/CPOE%20Fact%20Sheet.pdf.

LeFever, G. B. "Chasing Zero Events of Harm: An Urgent Call to Expand Safety Culture Work and Patient Engagement." *Nursing and Patient Care* (February 2010). http://www.yoursls.com/ConnectingHospitals-Communities.pdf.

———. "Issue Brief: Increased Use of Psychiatric Drugs in American Schools." Arlington, VA: The Lexington Institute, 2002.

LeFever, G. B., K. Allen, and E. A. Plasden. "Piloting a School-Wide Behavioral Intervention Study." In *132nd Annual Meeting of the American Public Health Association*. Washington, DC, 2004.

LeFever, G. B., A. P. Arcona, and D. O. Antonuccio. "ADHD among American Schoolchildren: Evidence of Overdiagnosis and Overuse of Medication." *Scientific Review of Mental Health Practice* 2, no. 1 (2003): 49–60.

LeFever, G. B., F. D. Butterfoss, and N. Vislocky. "High Prevalence of Attention Deficit Hyperactivity Disorder: Catalyst for Development of a School Health Coalition." *Family and Community Health* 22, no. 1 (1999): 38–49.

LeFever, G. B., K. V. Dawson, and A. L. Morrow. "The Extent of Drug Therapy for Attention-Deficit/Hyperactivity Disorder among Children in Public Schools." *American Journal of Public Health* 89, no. 9 (1999): 1359–64.

LeFever, G. B., J. L. Parker, A. L. Morrow, and M. S. Villers. "Understanding ADHD Issues in a Community with a High ADHD Prevalence Rate: Parent, Teacher, and Provider Perspectives." In *128th Annual Meeting of the American Public Health Association*. Boston, MA, 2000.

LeFever, G. B., M. S. Villers, A. L. Morrow, and E. S. Vaughn. "Parental Perceptions of Adverse Educational Outcomes among Children Diagnosed with ADHD: A Call for Improved School/Provider Collaboration." *Psychology in the Schools* 39, no. 1 (2002): 63–71.

Leonard, M., S. Graham, and D. Bonacum. "The Human Factor: The Critical Importance of Effective Teamwork and Communication in Providing Safe Care." *Quality and Safety in Health Care* 13, no. Suppl 1 (2004): 85–90.

Levinson, Daniel R. "Adverse Events in Skilled Nursing Facilities: National Incidence among Medicare Beneficiaries." Washington, DC: Department of Health and Human Services, 2014.

Liang, Stephen Y., Daniel L. Theodoro, Jeremiah D. Schuur, and Jonas Marschall. "Infection Prevention in the Emergency Department." *Infectious Disease* 64, no. 3 (2014): 299–313.

Liao, Joshua M., Eric J. Thomas, and Sigall K. Bell. "Speaking up About the Dangers of the Hidden Curriculum." *Health Affairs* 33, no. 1 (2014): 168–71.

Lucien Leape Institute. "Unmet Needs: Teaching Physicians to Provide Safe Patient Care." Boston, MA: National Patient Safety Foundation, 2010.

Lyons-Weiler, James. Chapter 6: Overdiagnosis of ADHD. In *Cures vs. Profits: Successes in Translational Research*. London: World Scientific, 2016.

Mack, K. M., C. S. Kelly, and A. L. Morrow. "Head Start: A Setting for Asthma Outreach and Prevention." *Family and Community Health* 22, no. 1 (1999): 28–37.

Mackay, Alan L. *A Dictionary of Scientific Quotations*. London: CRC Press, 1991, 219.

Makani, Hemadri. "Mark the Site Campaign." In *Success in Healthcare*, 2012.

Makary, Martin A., and Michael Daniel. "Medical Error—the Third Leading Cause of Death in the US." *BMJ* 353.

Makary, Martin A., Arnab Mukherjee, J. Bryan Sexton, Dora Syin, Emmanuelle Goodrich, Emily Hartmann, Lisa C. Rowen et al. "Operating Room Briefings and Wrong-Site Surgery." *Journal of the American College of Surgery* 204, no. 236–243 (2007).

Margolin, Frances S. "Getting to Zero: Reducing Rates of Clabsi in Community Hospitals." (2011). http://www.leapfroggroup.org/media/file/Final _GettingToZero.pdf.

Martinez, J. "What a Mess, Baby." *Daily News*, March 22, 2007.

Maurer, Maureen, Pam Dardess, Kristin L. Carman, Karen Frazier, and Lauren Smeeding. "Guide to Parent and Family Engagement: Environmental Scan Report." In *AHRQ Publication No. 12-0042-EF*. Rockville, MD: Agency for Healthcare Research and Quality, 2012.

McArdle, Megan. *The Up Side of Down: Why Failing Well Is the Key to Success.* New York: Penquin Books, 2015.

McCloskey, D. J., M. A. McDonald, J. Cook, S. Heurtin-Roberts, S. Updegrove, D. Smapson, S. Gutter, and M. Eder. "Community Engagement: Definitions and Organizing Concepts from the Literature." Edited by Public Health Practice Program Office. Atlanta, GA: Centers for Disease Control and Prevention, 2015.

McGlynn, Elizabeth A., Steven M. Asch, John Adams, Joan Keesey, Jennifer Hicks, Alison DeCristofaro, and Eve A. Kerr. "The Quality of Health Care Delivered to Adults in the United States." *New England Journal of Medicine* 348, no. 26 (2003): 2635–45.

McGuckin, M., R. Waterman, J. Storr, I. C. J. W. Bowler, M. Ashby, K. Topley, and L. Porten. "Evaluation of a Patient-Empowering Hand Hygiene Programme in the UK." *Journal of Hospital Infection* 48, no. 3 (2001): 222–27.

McNamara, S. A. "Incivility in Nursing: Unsafe Nurse, Unsafe Patients." *AORN Journal* 95, no. 4 (2012): 535–40.

Medical News Today. "Record 4.02 Billion Prescriptions in the United States in 2011." *MNT*, September 14, 2012. http://www.medicalnewstoday.com/releases/250213.php.

Mello, Michelle M., Richard C. Boothman, Timothy McDonald, Jeffrey Driver, Alan Lembitz, Darren Bouwmeester, Benjamin Dunlap, and Thomas Gallagher. "Communication-and-Resolution Programs: The Challenges and Lessons Learned from Six Early Adopters." *Health Affairs* 33, no. 1 (2014): 20–29.

Mello, Michelle M., Susan K. Senecal, Yelena Kuznetsov, and Janet S. Cohn. "Implementing Hospital-Based Communication-and-Resolution Programs: Lessons Learned in New York City." *Health Affairs* 33, no. 1 (2014): 30–36.

Mendelson, Dan, Rajeev Ramchand, Richard Abramson, and Anne Tumlinson. "Prescription Drugs in Nursing Homes: Managing Costs and Quality in a Complex Environment." In *NHPF Issue Brief.* National Health Policy Forum, 2002.

Mercer, Larry, Philip Felt, and Noell R. Snider. "Getting the Most out of Your Epic EMR Training Program." *White Paper* (2012). http://divurgent.com/wp-content/uploads/pdf/EpicEMRTrainingProgram.pdf.

Michaels, Robert K., Martin A. Makary, Yasser Dahab, Frank J. Frassica, Eugenie Heitmiller, Lisa C. Rowen, Richard Crotreau, Henry Brem, and Peter J. Pronovost. "Achieving the National Quality Forum's 'Never Events': Prevention of Wrong Site, Wrong Procedure, and Wrong Patient Operations." *Annals of Surgery* 245, no. 4 (2007): 526–32.

Monash Institute of Health Service Research. "Literature Review Regarding Patient Engagement in Patient Safety Initiatives." (2008). http://www
.safetyandquality.gov.au/wp-content/uploads/2012/01/Literature-Review
-Regarding-Patient-Engagement-in-Patient-Safety-Initiatives.pdf.

Moore, T. J., M. R. Cohen, and C. D. Furberg. "Serious Adverse Drug Events Reported to the Food and Drug Administration, 1998–2005." *Archives of Internal Medicine* 167, no. 16 (2007): 1752–59.

Morales, Tatiana. "Switched before Birth." (2004). August 4, 2004. http://www
.cbsnews.com/news/switched-before-birth/.

National Patient Safety Agency. "Health Literacy: Statistics at-a-Glance." April 2011. https://c.ymcdn.com/sites/www.npsf.org/resource/collection/9220B314
-9666-40DA-89DA-9F46357530F1/AskMe3_Stats_English.pdf.

———. "National Agenda for Action: Patients and Families in Patient Safety—Nothing About Me, without Me." https://c.ymcdn.com/sites/www.npsf
.org/resource/collection/ABAB3CA8-4E0A-41C5-A480-6DE8B793536C/
Nothing_About_Me.pdf.

———. "Safety Is Personal: Partnering with Patients and Families for the Safest Care." Boston, MA: National Patient Safety Foundation, 2014.

———. "Wristbands for Hospital Inpatients Improves Safety." http://www
.nrls.npsa.nhs.uk/EasySiteWeb/getresource.axd?AssetID=60032.

National Patient Safety Foundation. http://www.npsf.org/?page=aboutus.

National Public Radio. "Atul Gawande's 'Checklist' for Surgery Success." *Morning Edition*, January 5, 2010. http://www.npr.org/templates/story/
story.php?storyId=122226184.

Novack, D. H., R. Plumer, R. L. Smith, H. Ochitill, G. R. Morrow, and J. M. Bennett. "Changes in Physicians' Attitudes toward Telling the Cancer Patient." *JAMA* 241, no. 9 (1979): 897–900.

Occupational Safety and Health Administration. "Worker Safety in Your Hospital." OSHA. https://www.osha.gov/dsg/hospitals/documents/1.1_Data_
highlights_508.pdf.

Okuyama, Ayako, Cordula Wagner, and Bart Bijnen. "Speaking up for Patient Safety by Hospital-Based Health Care Professionals: A Literature Review." *BMC Health Services Research* 14 (2014): 61.

Parker, Stacy. "Health Care Hero Awards: Corporate Achievements in Health Care." *Inside Business*, February 17, 2012.

Pascale, Richard, Jerry Sternin, and Monique Sternin. *The Power of Positive Deviance: How Unlikely Innovators Solve the World's Toughest Problems.* Boston, MA: Harvard Business Press, 2010.

Pines, Jesse M., John J. Kelly, Helmut Meisl, James J. Augustine, Robert I. Broida, John R. Clarker, Heather Farley et al. "Procedural Safety in Emergency Care: A Conceptual Model and Recommendations." *Joint Commission Journal on Quality and Patient Safety* 38, no. 11 (2012): 516–26.

PR Newswire. "Boston Medical Center Teams up with Rhode Island Hospital, CVS Health to Address Use of Pharmacy-Based Naloxone to Combat Opioid Addiction and Overdoses." news release, 2015. http://www.prnewswire.com/news-releases/boston-medical-center-teams-up-with-rhode-island-hospital-cvs-health-to-address-use-of-pharmacy-based-naloxone-to-combat-opioid-addiction-and-overdoses-300124914.html.

Pratt, Sephen, Linda Kenney, Susan D. Scott, and Albert W. Wu. "How to Develop a Second Victim Support Program: A Toolkit for Health Care Organizations." *Joint Commission Journal on Quality and Patient Safety* 38, no. 5 (2012): 235–40.

Pronovost, Peter J., Christine A. Goeschel, Elizabeth Colantuoni, Sam Watson, Lisa H. Lubomski, Sean M. Berenholtz, David A. Thompson et al. "Sustaining Reductions in Catheter Related Bloodstream Infections in Michigan Intensive Care Units: Observational Study." *BMJ: British Medical Journal* 340 (2010): c309.

Pronovost, Peter, Dale Needham, Sean Berenholtz, David Sinopoli, Haitao Chu, Sara Cosgrove, Bryan Sexton et al. "An Intervention to Decrease Catheter-Related Bloodstream Infections in the ICU." *New England Journal of Medicine* 355, no. 26 (2006): 2725–32.

Pronovost, P. J., and E. Vohr. *Safe Patients, Smart Hospitals: How One Doctor's Checklist Can Help Us Change Health Care from the Inside Out.* New York: Penquin Group, 2010.

Quinones, Sam. *Dreamland: The True Tale of America's Opiate Epidemic.* Dexter, MI: Bloomsbury Press, 2015.

Radley, David C., Melanie R. Wasserman, Lauren E. W. Olsho, Sarah J. Shoemaker, Mark D. Spranca, and Bethany Bradshaw. "Reduction in Medication Errors in Hospitals Due to Adoption of Computerized Provider Order Entry Systems." *Journal of the American Medical Informatics Association* 20, no. 3 (2013): 470–76.

Reason, James. "Human Error: Models and Management." *BMJ: British Medical Journal* 320, no. 7237 (2000): 768–70.

Reinertsen, James L., Michael D. Bisgnano, and Maureen Pugh. *Seven Leadership Leverage Points for Organizational-Level Improvement in Health Care.* Cambridge, MA: Institute for Healthcare Improvement, 2008.

Reising, Deanna L., and Patricia N. Allen. "Protecting Yourself from Malpractice Claims." *American Nurse Today* (February 2007): 39–44.

Revere, Audrey. "JCAHO National Patient Safety Goals for 2007." *Topics in Patient Safety* 7, no. 1 (2007).

Ring, David C., James H. Herndon, and Gregg S. Meyer. "Case 34-2010." *New England Journal of Medicine* 363, no. 20 (2010): 1950–57.

Robbins, Alexandra. *The Nurses: A Year of Secrets, Drama, and Miracles with the Heroes of the Hospital.* New York: Workman Publishing Company, Inc., 2015.

Rosenstein, A. H., and M. O'Daniel. "A Survey of the Impact of Disruptive Behaviors and Communication Defects on Patient Safety." *Joint Commission Journal on Quality and Patient Safety* 34, no. 8 (2008): 464–71.

Rosenstock, I. M., V. J. Stretcher, and M. H. Becker. "Social Learning Theory and the Health Belief Model." *Health Education Quarterly* 15, no. 2 (1988): 175–83.

Rubin, G. *Better Than Before: Mastering the Habits of Our Everyday Lives.* New York: Crown Publishers, 2015.

Saad, Karim. "Discovery & Action Dialogues: A Tool for Getting Started." In *SharedCare: Partners for Patients*, edited by BC Patient Safety & Quality Council, 2013.

Sack, K. "A Hospital Hand-Washing Project to Save Lives and Money." *New York Times*, September 10 2009.

Sandars, John, and Gary Cook. *ABC of Patient Safety.* Malden, MA: Blackwell Publishing, 2007.

Schwarz, A. "Drowned in a Stream of Prescriptions." *New York Times*, February 2 2013.

———. "The Selling of Attention Deficit Disorder." *New York Times*, December 14 2013.

Scott, R. "The Direct Medical Costs of Healthcare-Associated Infections in U.S. Hospitals and the Benefits of Prevention." Centers for Disease Control and Prevention, 2009.

Scott, Susan D. "The 'Second Victim' Phenomenon: A Harsh Reality of Health Care Professions." *Perpectives on Safety* (May 2011). https://psnet. ahrq.gov/perspectives/perspective/102.

Shannon, Sarah E., Mary Beth Foglia, Mary Hardy, and Thomas H. Gallagher. "Disclosing Errors to Patients: Perspectives of Registered Nurses." *The Joint Commission Journal on Quality and Patient Safety* 35, no. 1 (2009): 5–12.

Shekelle, P. G., R. M. Wachter, P. J. Pronovost, K. Schoelles, K. M. McDonald, S. M. Dy, K. Shojania, et al. "Making Health Care Safer II: An Updated Critical Analysis of the Evidence for Patient Safety Practices." In *Comparative Effectiveness Review No. 211*, edited by Southern California-RAND Evidence-based Practice Cneter. Rockville, MD: Agency for Healthcare Research and Quality, 2013.

Sickbert-Bennett, E. E., L. M. Dibiase, W. Schade, E. S. Wolak, D. J. Weber, and W. A. Rutala. "Reduction of Healthcare-Associated Infections by Exceeding High Compliance with Hand Hygiene Practices." *Emerging Infectious Diseases* 22, no. 9 (2016): 1628–30.

Sidorov, J. "It Ain't Necessarily So: The Electronic Health Record and the Unlikely Prospect of Reducing Health Care Costs: Much of the Literature on EHRS Fails to Support the Primary Rationales for Using Them." *Health Affairs* 25, no. 4 (2006): 1079–85.

Simpson, Elizabeth. "Va. Beach Psychiatrist's License to Be Suspended." *Virginian-Pilot*, October 28, 2014.

Singhal, Arvind, and Karen Greiner. "Do What You Can with What You Have, Where You Are Now: A Quest to Eliminate MRSA at the Va Pittsburgh Healthcare System." *Deeper Learning* 1, no. 4 (2007): 1–12.

Smiley, Kim. "The Willie King Case: Wrong Foot Amputated." In *Patient Safety Blog*, 2014.

Smith, George David, and Frederick Dalzell. *Wisdom from the Robber Barons: Enduring Lessons from Rockefeller, Morgan, and the First Industrialists*. New York: Basic Books, 2000.

Sorra, J., T. Famolaro, N. Dyer, D. Nelson, and S. C. Smith. "Hospital Survey on Patient Safety Culture." Rockville, MD: Agency for Healthcare Research and Quality, 2012.

Stahel, P. F., A. L. Sabel, M. S. Victoroff, et al. "Wrong-Site and Wrong-Patient Procedures in the Universal Protocol Era: Analysis of a Prospective Database of Physician Self-Reported Occurrences." *Archives of Surgery* 145, no. 10 (2010): 978–84.

Studdert, David M., Michelle M. Mello, and Troyen A. Brennan. "Medical Malpractice." *New England Journal of Medicine* 350, no. 3 (2004): 283–92.

Studdert, David M., Michelle M. Mello, Atul A. Gawande, Tejal K. Gandhi, Allen Kachalia, Catherine Yoon, Ann Louise Puopolo, and Troyen A. Brennan. "Claims, Errors, and Compensation Payments in Medical Malpractice Litigation." *New England Journal of Medicine* 354, no. 19 (2006): 2024–33.

Substance Abuse and Mental Health Service Administration. "Results from the 2013 National Survey on Drug Use and Health: Summary of National Findings." Substance Abuse and Mental Health Service Administration. Rockville, MD, 2014.

Tartt, Donna. *The Goldfinch*. New York: Little, Brown and Company, 2013.

Tobias, Dianne E., and Mark Sey. "General and Psychotherapeutic Medication Use in 328 Nursing Facilities: A Year 2000 National Survey." *Consultant Pharmacist* 16, no. 1 (2001): 52.

United Nations Office on Drugs and Crime. "Word Drug Report 2012." http://www.unodc.org/unodc/en/data-and-analysis/WDR-2012.html.

Van Den Bos, Jill, Karan Rustagi, Travis Gray, Michael Halford, Eva Ziemkie-wicz, and Jonathan Shreve. "The $17.1 Billion Problem: The Annual Cost of Measurable Medical Errors." *Health Affairs* 30, no. 4 (2011): 596–603.

van der Sijs, Heleen, Jos Aarts, Arnold Vulto, and Marc Berg. "Overriding of Drug Safety Alerts in Computerized Physician Order Entry." *Journal of the American Medical Informatics Association : JAMIA* 13, no. 2 (March–April 2006): 138–47.

Van Kanegan, G., and M. Boyette. *How to Survive Your Hospital Stay: The Complete Guide to Getting the Care You Need—and Avoiding Problems You Don't.* New York: Fireside, 2003.

Varjavand, N., S. Nair, and E. Gracely. "A Call to Address the Curricular Provision of Emotional Support in the Event of Medical Errors and Adverse Events." *Medical Education* 46 (2012): 1149–51.

Visser, S. N., M. L. Danielson, R. H. Bitsko, J. R. Holbrook, M. D. Kogan, R. M. Ghandour, R. Perou, and S. J. Blumberg. "Trends in the Parent-Report of Health Care Provider-Diagnosed and Medicated Attention-Deficit/ Hyperactivity Disorder: United States, 2003–2011." *Journal of the American Academy of Child & Adolescent Psychiatry* (2013).

Voepel-Lewis, T., E. Pechlavanidis, C. Burke, and A. Talsma. "Nursing Sur-veillance Moderates the Relationship between Staffing Levels and Pediatric Postoperative Serious Adverse Events: A Nested-Case Control Study." *International Journal of Nursing Studies* 50, no. 7 (2012): 905–13.

Wachter, R. M. "Is the Patient Safety Movement in Danger of Flickering Out?" In *Wachter's World*, edited by R. M. Wachter, 2013.

Wachter, Robert. *The Digital Doctor: Hope, Hype, and Harm at the Dawn of Medicine's Computer Age.* New York: McGraw-Hill, 2015.

Wandersman, A., and J. Alderman. "Community Interventions and Effective Prevention." *American Psychologist* 58 (2003): 441–48.

Ware, Mark, and Michael Mabe. "The STM Report: An Overview of Scien-tific and Scholarly Publishing." In *The STM Report*. Netherlands, 2012.

Waterman, Amy D., Thomas H. Gallagher, Jane Garbutt, Brian M. Waterman, Victoria Fraser, and Thomas E. Burroughs. "Brief Report: Hospitalized Patients' Attitudes About and Participation in Error Prevention." *Journal of General Internal Medicine* 21, no. 4 (2006): 367–70.

Watson, Gretchen LeFever. "The Deadly Dangers of ADHD Drugs." *Virginian-Pilot*, October 2, 2016.

———. "The Hospital Safety Crisis: Unifying Efforts of Healthcare Systems, Public Health, and Society." *Society* 53, no. 4 (2016): 1–7.

Watson, G. L., and A. P. Arcona. "8 Ways to Respond to Student ADHD Drug Abuse." *Campus Safety* (2014): 34–37.

————. "ADHD Drug Abuse Epidemic Prompts New School Rules." *Campus Safety*, May 3, 2014.

Watson, Gretchen LeFever, Andrea Powell Arcona, and David O. Antonuccio. "The ADHD Drug Abuse Crisis on American College Campuses." *Ethical Human Psychology and Psychiatry* 17, no. 1 (2015): 5–21.

Watson, Gretchen LeFever, Andrea Powell Arcona, David O. Antonuccio, and D. Healy. "Shooting the Messenger: The Case of ADHD." *Journal of Contemporary Psychotherapy* 44, no. 1 (2014): 43–52.

Weems, Carolyn. "Fighting Heroin in Virginia Beach." *Virginian-Pilot*, November 20, 2015.

Weiser, Thomas G., Scott E. Regenbogen, Katherine D. Thompson, Alex B. Haynes, Stuart R. Lipsitz, William R. Berry, and Atul A. Gawande. "An Estimation of the Global Volume of Surgery: A Modelling Strategy Based on Available Data." *The Lancet* 372, no. 9633 (2008): 139–44.

Whatis.com. "Workaround." http://whatis.techtarget.com/definition/work around.

World Health Organization. "Patient Identification." *Patient Safety Solutions* 1, 2 (2007). http://www.who.int/patientsafety/solutions/patientsafety/PS -Solution2.pdf.

————. "WHO Guidelines for Safe Surgery (First Edition)." Geneva, Switzerland: World Health Organization, 2008.

————. "WHO Guidelines on Hand Hygiene in Health Care: A Summary." Geneva, Switzerland: World Health Organization, 2009.

Wu, Albert W. *Being Open with Patients and Families About Adverse Events.* Podcast audio. Medical Center Hour Being Open with Patients and Families, 2010. https://www.youtube.com/watch?v=DkYm8HFq_Vk.

————. "Medical Error: The Second Victim: The Doctor Who Makes the Mistake Needs Help Too." *BMJ: British Medical Journal* 320, no. 7237 (2000): 726–27.

Wu, Albert W., Dennis J. Boyle, Gordon Wallace, and Kathleen M. Mazor. "Disclosure of Adverse Events in the United States and Canada: An Update, and a Proposed Framework for Improvement." *Journal of Public Health Research* 2, no. 3 (2013): e32.

Zhong, Wenjun, Hilal Maradit-Kremers, Jennifer L. St. Sauver, Barbara P. Yawn, Jon O. Ebbert, Véronique L. Roger, Debra J. Jacobson, et al. "Age and Sex Patterns of Drug Prescribing in a Defined American Population." *Mayo Clinic* 88, no. 7 (2013): 697–707.

Zimmerman, T., and G. Amori. "The Silent Organizational Pathology of Insidious Intimidation." *Journal of Healthcare Risk Management* 30, no. 3 (2011): 5–6, 8–15.

Index

23, 42; practitioners, 4, 139; research, 23

Quinones, Sam, 104

Reason, James, 30
Regan, Brian, 43
Reinertsen, James L., 133
retrofitted shame, 35–36
Ring, David, 64
ripple effect, 9, 136. *See also* secondary victim
Robbins, Alexandra, 107
root cause, 16
Rubin, Gretchen, 33

safety as a core value, 16
safety culture, ix, 2, 15–17, 43, 50
safety versus quality, 16
Santillan, Jesica, 62, 77
School Health Initiative for Education (SHINE), 124–127
Schrodinger, Erwin, 7
scripted language, 154–155
second victim, 136, 138. *See also* ripple effect
Semmelweis, Ignaz, 48–49, 77
sentinel event, 66
shame. *See* retrofitted shame
sharp vs. blunt end of care, 144–145
Sign Your Site Campaign, 66
slips and lapses, 4, 32, 96
social norms, 117
Southeastern Virginia. See Hampton Roads
speak up for safety, 3, 40–42, 69, 72
spell check factor, 54, 143
staffing, 145
Standards of Learning tests, 125

Sternin, Jerry and Monique, 116–119
Stewart, Jan, 107
sticky message, 55, 58, 81, 111
stimulus funding, 17
superbugs, 45–46. *See* healthcare-associated infection
surgical errors, 65. *See also* off-the-mark procedure; *see also* trifecta
The Swiss Cheese Model, 30–33, 54, 67, 86, 96, 145
system error/issue, 10, 96

team huddle, 72
Tobacco Master Settlement Agreement, 131
To Err is Human, 1–2, 13–15, 87, 136, 155
tragedy of the commons, 34–35
training:
  patient: 4, 36–42
  provider: 4, 11–23, 18, 36, 76–77, 148, 153–154
transparency, 15, 132
trifecta, 3–4, 22–23, 25–28, 42

United in Safety, 113–114
Universal Protocol, 70–81,

VA Health Care System, 152
Veterans Administration, 13
Veteran's Administration Pittsburgh Healthcare System, 119–121
Virginia, 108, 125
Virginia Beach, Virginia, 104, 108, 124. *See also* Hampton Roads, Virginia.
Virginia Beach City Public Schools, 108, 126

About the Author

Gretchen LeFever Watson, PhD, graduated from Boston University, *summa cum laude* and with distinction in psychology. She earned a doctorate in clinical and developmental psychology from the University of Illinois, Chicago, and completed postdoctoral training in pediatric psychology at Georgetown University Medical School. Mid-career, she received intensive training in the science of safety from nuclear power engineers and national healthcare leaders.

As a clinical psychologist who has worked in academic, healthcare, and business settings for over 20 years, Dr. Watson is passionate about improving the health and safety of individuals, companies, and communities. She was among the first to document drug overtreatment for ADHD in the United States and to demonstrate that disruptive conduct can be successfully reduced through schoolwide behavioral interventions. She has appeared on national TV and radio programs such as *CNN Headline News,* the *PBS News Hour, and The Diane Rehm Show.* Her work has been published in an array of scientific journals and has been discussed in popular magazines, including *Psychology Today, Science, Popular Science,* and *The Weekly Standard* as well as newspapers across the United States and in Europe.

More recently, Dr. Watson received the Healthcare Hero award from *Inside Business* for her work in patient safety, graduated from Virginia's CIVIC Leadership Institute, and was included in a prestigious list of 100 international scientists recognized by the *British Medical Journal* for their unbiased reviews of health research. She also received the *Superintendent's Quality Award* from one of the nation's largest school districts for her innovative teacher training program that demonstrated improvements in student behavior and learning. She is President of Safety & Leadership Solutions, a consulting firm for organizational safety and change management. Spending time with her daughter and windsurfing with her husband and friends around the world are two of her favorite things to do. She can be reached through her website: drgretchenwatson.com.